PHYSICAL THERAPY PHARMACOLOGY

Physical Therapy Pharmacology

LYNNE EDDY, Ph.D., P.T.

Long Beach, California
Formerly:
Associate Professor
Department of Physical Therapy
University of Southern California
Los Angeles, California

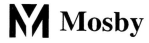 **Mosby**

A Harcourt Health Sciences Company
St. Louis London Philadelphia Sydney Toronto

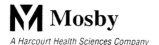
A Harcourt Health Sciences Company

Sponsoring Editor: David K. Marshall
Assistant Editor: Julie Tryboski
Assistant Director, Manuscript Services: Frances M. Perveiler
Project Supervisor: Carol A. Reynolds
Proofroom Manager: Barbara Kelly

Mosby, Inc.
11830 Westline Industrial Drive
St. Louis, MO 63146

3 4 5 6 7 8 9 0 CA PP 96

Library of Congress Cataloging-in-Publication Data
Eddy, Lynne.
    Physical therapy pharmacology / Lynne Eddy.
      p. cm.
    Includes bibliographical references and index.
    ISBN 0-8151-3076-7
    1. Pharmacology. 2. Drugs—Side effects. 3. Physical therapy.
  I. Title.
    [DNLM: 1. Pharmacology. 2. Physical Therapy. QV 4 E21p]
RM301.E33 1991   91-38913
615′.1—dc20
DNLM/DLC

PREFACE

This book is an overview of therapeutic agents commonly used by patients seen in the practice of physical therapy. Specifically stressed are drugs affecting the cardio-vascular-renal, nervous, respiratory, endocrine, and gastrointestinal systems. Medical reasons for the drug treatment, specific actions of the therapeutic agents, and adverse effects are the main focus. Problems related to polypharmacy, especially in the geriatric population, are emphasized as needed. This book covers pharmacologic treatment of chronic medical conditions. Antibiotics specifically are omitted from this book: while they do have important side effects, their use is generally of an acute (10-day) treatment duration. This book is directed to physical therapy students at any level, baccalaureate, certificate, or graduate, and to the practicing clinician. No pharmacology background is assumed. A working knowledge of physiology and path-ophysiology is expected; however, pathophysiology may be taught concurrently with pharmacology. The goal of this book is to acquaint the physical therapist with drug actions that may affect physical therapy treatment.

My 10 years of teaching pharmacology to physical therapy students constitutes the background for this book. I think it is important to know one major drug from each class of drugs, so I have attempted to present the prototypical drug or the most commonly used drug from each class. Other drugs and doses are listed for information purposes only. Because physical therapists do not prescribe drugs, there is no reason to learn the doses. I have included both generic and trade names. Certain drugs are more frequently referred to by their trade names, while others are referred to by their generic names.

Lynne Eddy, Ph.D., P.T.

CONTENTS _____

PART I

Introduction to Pharmacology

Chapter 1

General Concepts

Pharmacology is the study of drugs. A **drug** is any chemical agent that affects living processes; for our purposes, a drug is used to prevent or alter disease processes. A drug does not initiate cellular actions, but rather modifies—either stimulates or depresses—biochemical or physiologic functional capabilities of the cell. It can mimic actions of endogenous substances or can interfere with actions of endogenous substances.

Drug names are at three levels. The first is the **chemical name**, which defines the chemical structure. This name is rarely used in medical practice. The **generic** or **nonproprietary name** is the common name given to a drug by the United States Adopted Names Council. **Proprietary** or **trademark** names are given to a drug by a specific pharmaceutical company. When a company receives a patent for a particular drug, only that company may market the drug under its own trade name. Patent rights are for 17 years from the patent approval date. If a drug is marketed by more than one company, it will have more than one proprietary name. Combinations of drugs will have separate proprietary names for each mixture.

In the United States, the Food and Drug Administration (FDA) has the authority to approve drugs for human use. After preclinical (animal) and clinical (human) testing for both safety and efficacy, a pharmaceutical company submits a new drug application to the FDA. The FDA approves a drug for specific indications. However, a physician may prescribe an approved drug for other than designated indications. This use of a drug for unapproved indications yields clinical data that the FDA can review. Possibly the new indication will then be approved by the FDA also. Other countries have similar mechanisms for approving drugs for human use. Each country has developed its own guidelines; therefore, a drug may be approved in one country but not in others.

Pharmacology can be divided into two major divisions: pharmacokinetics and pharmacodynamics.

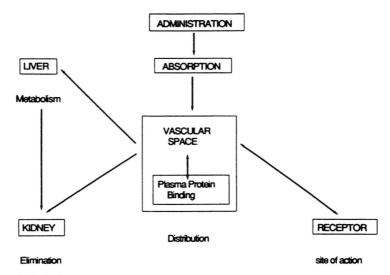

FIG 1–1
Schematic diagram of the basic compartments of pharmacokinetics, from administration to elimination, shows distribution of a drug by the blood to the site of action, site of metabolism, and site of elimination.

PHARMACOKINETICS

Pharmacokinetics encompasses all the processes involved in transport of the drug to its target site and removal of the drug and its metabolites from the body. These processes include absorption from its site of administration, distribution within the body to the tissues, metabolism to more active or inactive products, and excretion of drugs and metabolites, or *how the body acts upon a drug*. This involves active and passive transport across membranes, protein binding, and enzymatic reactions to the drug. The different aspects of pharmacokinetics are depicted graphically in Figure 1–1.

Absorption

Drugs must pass through lipid membranes to enter the blood stream subsequent to all routes of administration other than intravenous. The lipid solubility of a drug increases its rate of transfer across the membranes. Drugs can be administered by any one of a number of routes.

1. Oral administration is the most common, the most convenient, and generally the most economical method of drug administration. However, certain drugs cannot be administered orally. These include proteins, which are degraded by intestinal proteases, and those chemicals not absorbed from the intestinal tract, either because they are metabolized by intestinal bacteria or form nonabsorbable complexes. Drugs

that are effective after oral administration are absorbed through the intestinal epithelium and enter the blood vessels of the intestinal tract. They are then carried directly to the liver by the hepatic portal system. If a drug is rapidly metabolized by the liver, then little will actually enter the systemic circulation. This is referred to as the **"first-pass effect."** Thus, even if a drug is well absorbed, its plasma concentration may be decreased because of this first-pass effect. In order to bypass the first-pass effect, drugs may be administered by another route that permits the drug to enter the systemic circulation but avoids first-pass degradation in the liver. Examples of administration routes that prevent first-pass metabolism are intravenous, intramuscular, and sublingual. Also, changes in chemical structure may alter the liver metabolism but have no effect on the drug action.

Frequently, chemists can alter the chemical structure of a drug to reduce the first-pass metabolism. This allows more of the drug to reach the systemic circulation. **Timed release** or **sustained release** formulations are designed to produce slow, uniform dissolution of the administered product, allowing for prolonged absorption of the drug, up to 8 hours or more. This can allow for overnight maintenance of adequate blood levels of the drug without the patient having to wake up to take another dose. However, variable dissolution may lead to erratic release of the drug. Constant therapeutic blood levels may be difficult to maintain. **Enteric coated tablets** are designed such that the outer coat is acid resistant, but readily dissolves in the alkaline pH of the intestine. This may be of an advantage for drugs that may irritate the stomach but are absorbed in the intestinal tract. This formulation may also be used to protect drugs that are degraded in the acid environment of the stomach but can be absorbed in the small intestine.

2. Intravenous injection provides the quickest onset of action; however, the drug must be in an aqueous solution. This method is difficult to self-administer. Intramuscular or subcutaneous injection routes are more easily managed than intravenous, and the drug does not have to be in aqueous solution. Formulations can be such that absorption from the intramuscular or subcutaneous injection site is prolonged, for example, suspensions in oil.

3. The sublingual route offers the advantage of fairly rapid absorption and onset of action. Because of venous drainage, drugs taken sublingually bypass the liver and avoid "first-pass metabolism." This route is appropriate for drugs that can be absorbed through the mucous membranes of the oral cavity.

4. Topical administration is appropriate for treatment of localized epidermal areas, such as skin or mucous membranes. Generally, topical administration avoids systemic effects of the drug; however, sometimes the drug is absorbed through the skin and systemic effects occur. Certain superficial eye diseases may be treated by the topical approach. Oral inhalation of drugs used to treat respiratory diseases is a method of topical administration. A drug administered by this manner has direct accessibility to the airways and, with little systemic absorption, there are few side effects.

The transdermal approach is a topical route also used for certain drugs that can be absorbed through the skin to treat systemic diseases. Adhesive skin patches are impregnated with the drug, and the dose administered is proportional to the size of the patch.

Distribution

Distribution of a drug to the different tissues depends on blood flow. The heart, liver, kidney, and brain receive greater blood flow than do muscle, viscera, skin, and adipose tissue. However, all drugs do not gain access to the central nervous system, in spite of its blood flow. Entry of drugs into either the extracellular space of the central nervous system or the cerebrospinal fluid is restricted because of the tight junctions between the endothelial cells of the capillaries. This architectural feature is known as the "blood-brain barrier." Lipid-soluble drugs are more likely to penetrate this barrier. The absorbed drug is distributed throughout the body into a **volume of distribution** (V_d). The volume of distribution is not a specific body fluid or volume, such as blood volume. Factors such as plasma protein binding and tissue binding govern distribution of the drug between plasma water, extracellular water, intracellular water, and total body water. Also, partitioning of the drug between water and fat (depending on the water/lipid solubility of the drug), and the effects of circulatory redistribution, alter the volume of distribution for a drug. **Bioavailability** refers to the amount of the drug that reaches its target of action. This is affected by gastrointestinal absorption, plasma protein binding, adipose tissue storage, biotransformation to other products, and elimination.

Binding of a drug to plasma proteins retains the drug within the vascular space. This binding prevents the drug from acting outside the vascular system, and also prevents its extravascular metabolism and excretion. Plasma protein binding by drugs is a reversible process and depends on the concentration of the drug and the affinity between the drug and the binding site. The concentration dependence follows the **Law of Mass Action**. Increasing the concentration of the drug causes an increase in the drug–plasma protein complex formation. Conversely, lowering the drug concentration leads to a decrease in the drug–plasma protein complex. The affinity, or tightness of binding, determines the ratio of bound to unbound drug at a given concentration. The "free" or unbound drug is the only form available to interact with its receptor, or to be metabolized. The drug that is complexed to the protein is not active and is essentially in a readily available storage. Thus, drugs that do not bind to plasma proteins generally have a quicker onset of action and a shorter duration of action than drugs that are heavily bound to plasma proteins.

There may be competition between drugs for plasma protein binding sites. This competition and subsequent displacement from the binding sites increases the free concentration of the drug displaced from the plasma protein, and may cause toxic reactions. Competition of drugs for binding sites on plasma proteins is responsible for many toxic reactions when more than one drug is administered. This does not necessarily mean that the drugs cannot be administered together, but doses and times of administration may have to be altered to prevent toxicity. Lipid-soluble drugs may be stored in adipose tissue, acting as a drug repository. This may cause a lower plasma concentration but a longer duration of action. Storage in fatty tissue is of concern in the obese, with an absolute increase in adipose tissue, and in the elderly when the ratio of body fat to lean body weight increases while the body weight remains the same.

Metabolism and Elimination

Enzymatic alteration of a drug, which is called biotransformation, may lead to the formation of a more active metabolite, to a less active or inactive metabolite, or to a toxic metabolite. The microsomal enzyme system in the liver is responsible for many drug biotransformations. Most microsomal enzyme reactions degrade a drug to more water-soluble end products, which are then excreted by the kidney. Volatile gases, such as the inhalation anesthetic agents, are mainly excreted from the body by the lungs. Some drugs are secreted with the bile into the intestinal tract, and can then either be reabsorbed or excreted with the feces. When a drug is reabsorbed from the intestinal tract and given a second chance to exert its effect, it is said to have undergone enterohepatic circulation. Some water-soluble drugs are filtered by the kidney and excreted as the intact drug.

The **elimination half-life** of a drug is the time in which the concentration of the drug falls to one-half of its original amount. This depends on plasma protein binding, liver metabolism, and kidney excretion. When repeated doses of a drug are given at regular intervals, the blood concentration will increase until an equilibrium is reached. At equilibrium the dose administered equals the amount eliminated. This equilibrium is referred to as the steady-state or plateau level. A drug administered at an interval close to its half-life requires about four to five administrations (half-lives) for steady state to be reached. If reaching the plateau in shorter time is desired, a higher dose can be administered initially. This is referred to as a **loading dose**. Steady-state levels are important in chronic drug therapy. At the steady-state level, plasma concentrations of the drug oscillate around the mean or average plasma concentration: that is, from the peak plasma level after administration of the drug to the minimum plasma level just before the next dose is administered. These maximum and minimum levels ("peaks and troughs") should be within the **therapeutic range**. The therapeutic range is defined as that below which the desired effect is usually not seen and above which toxic effects are seen. If these peaks and troughs of drug concentrations are outside the therapeutic range, an insufficient response may alternate with a toxic response. This is more of a problem with drugs that have short half-lives.

Some drugs have a duration of action that is longer than the plasma levels would indicate. This occurs through interaction of the drug with its receptor, initiating reactions that continue even without the presence of the drug. In these cases the **biologic half-life** is more important than the plasma concentration. Biologic half-life refers to the time of the response, rather than the plasma concentration.

PHARMACODYNAMICS

Pharmacodynamics includes the interaction of the active form of the drug with its site of action and initiation of processes resulting in the biological effect. This area of pharmacology is concerned with the biochemical and physiologic effects of a drug and its mechanism of action, or *how the drug acts upon the body*. This involves alteration of membrane properties, interaction with enzymes and receptors, and subsequent cellular reactions.

The site of action of a drug is where it produces its effect. This may be a specific organ system, or the drug may cause more generalized body effects. For a drug to have an action in the body, most must bind to a **receptor**. A receptor is a specific macromolecule (i.e., protein) that "recognizes" the drug. The receptor may be on the cell membrane or inside the cell. The binding of the drug to its specific receptor causes an activated complex which then triggers the cellular reactions. If the receptor is on the outside of the cell membrane, the formation of the activated complex sends a signal through the membrane, causing an action inside the cell. This is a mechanism by which a drug that cannot pass through the cell membrane can cause an intracellular action. The cellular response is frequently mediated by small molecular weight substances, which are called "second messengers." The second messenger may not be unique to a cell type, but is synthesized only in response to a particular drug-receptor complex. In many different cells adenosine $3':5' =$ cyclic phosphate (cyclic AMP) is the second messenger. However, its formation in a particular cell occurs only when a drug interacts with its specific receptor.

Generally, a drug binds to its receptor by a reversible mechanism. How much drug is bound to a receptor depends on the **affinity** of the drug for the receptor and the concentration of the drug. The concentration dependence follows the **Law of Mass Action**. Increasing the concentration of the drug causes an increase in the drug-receptor complex formation. Conversely, lowering the drug concentration leads to a decrease in the drug-receptor complex. The process of drug-receptor interaction is similar to the binding of a drug to plasma proteins; however, in the latter case, an action is not initiated. Also, a receptor is more specific for a particular drug than is the plasma protein binding site.

A drug that binds to a receptor and produces an action is referred to as an **agonist**. A drug that binds to a receptor and does not produce an action, but rather blocks another substance, endogenous or exogenous, from binding to that receptor is called an **antagonist** or blocker. Some drugs bind to a receptor and produce less of an effect than an agonist, and yet can prevent an agonist from binding. These are referred to as **partial agonists**. Partial agonists have properties of both agonists and antagonists.

A drug's **mechanism of action** is how it produces its effect at the cellular level. Drugs may alter membrane properties, changing ionic permeability or transport systems, alter enzyme activity, or alter synthesis of products, all of which are important to cellular processes.

The response to a drug depends on the dose of the drug. The higher the dose, the greater the response, to a maximum or ceiling effect. Dose-response curves are used to compare **potencies** of similarly acting drugs. Potency is the amount of drug needed to produce a certain effect. This is clinically unimportant, except if the effective dose requires taking of multiple pills at one time. The **efficacy** of a drug is the maximum response to a drug. This is clinically important.

A dose-response curve records the response to increasing concentrations of the drug. Plotting the responses to two drugs having the same type of response can

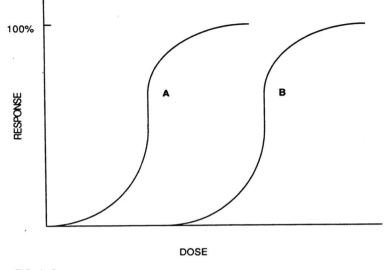

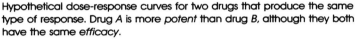

FIG 1–2
Hypothetical dose-response curves for two drugs that produce the same
type of response. Drug A is more *potent* than drug B, although they both
have the same *efficacy*.

show a comparison of potencies. In the example shown in Figure 1–2, both drugs
have the same efficacy, that is, the same maximum or ceiling effect. However, drug
A is more potent than drug B, in that a lower dose of drug A is needed to produce a
given level of response compared with drug B.

A time-concentration curve demonstrates the plasma concentration obtained
from a single administration of a drug (Fig 1–3). All aspects of pharmacokinetics
can alter the shape of this curve. An absolute decrease in absorption can decrease
the peak concentration. A displacement from plasma protein binding can cause an
increase in the peak concentration, but a shorter duration of action. An increase in
metabolism or elimination can decrease the area under the curve (AUC). Conversely, a decrease in metabolism or elimination can increase the area under the
curve. The time the drug remains above the therapeutic concentration is the duration of action.

The median effective dose, ED_{50}, is the dose that produces a specific response
in 50% of individuals. This is used to compare the potencies of similarly acting
drugs. The median lethal dose, LD_{50}, is the dose that is lethal to 50% of individuals.
The therapeutic index is the ratio of LD_{50} to ED_{50} and reflects the margin of safety
of a drug. A drug with a low therapeutic index has a therapeutic dose that is close to
its toxic dose. Thus, toxic reactions may be seen at doses near the therapeutic dose.

A drug does not produce only one effect. The intended medical effect of a drug
is defined as its **therapeutic effect**. A drug's **side effects** are not the intended medi-

cal effect, and are generally not harmful, but may be uncomfortable to some patients. The term **toxic effects** is generally reserved for those effects that are harmful. These may be an extension of the therapeutic or side effects, or totally unrelated. **Adverse effect** is the term frequently used to include both side effects and toxic effects. A **carcinogen** is a substance that produces cancer. A **teratogen** produces physical defects in the unfertilized ovum or sperm, or in the developing embryo. Many drugs can cross the placenta and, depending on the stage of pregnancy, interfere with normal fetal development. Generally, the first trimester is the most important for initial development of the fetal organ systems. However, many women do not know they are pregnant during this early developmental stage and may unknowingly be exposed to teratogenic drugs.

Certain biologic factors influence how a person responds to a drug. Although no two people are alike, individual differences may have little or no consequence in relation to pharmacokinetics or pharmacodynamics. However, the following factors may have sufficient effects on drug metabolism, action, and other responses to require a change in dose or drug:

1. *Age.* Children and the elderly are generally more susceptible to the actions of a drug. This may relate to activity of the metabolizing enzymes, the fat/lean ratio and distribution of drugs, or the rate of excretion of drugs and byproducts. Physiologic age-related changes may be responsible for alterations in drug response seen in the elderly. Age-related changes in pharmacokinetics are more commonly seen in the elderly. Tissue perfusion, except to the brain, decreases with age. In fact, the percent of cardiac output to the brain actually may increase with age. This may explain, in part, the greater sensitivity of the elderly to drugs that act on the central nervous system. Also, the liver shows some age-related changes, such as decreased total mass, decreased enzyme activity, and decreased hepatic blood flow. There is also

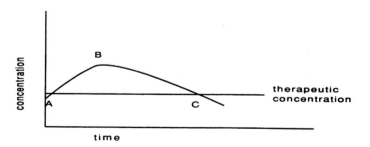

FIG 1–3

A hypothetical time-concentration curve. The area under the curve (AUC) is the time summation of the drug concentration above the therapeutic concentration. Point A is the onset of action, when the drug concentration rises to the therapeutic concentration. Point B is the peak concentration. At point C the drug concentration drops below the therapeutic concentration and there is insufficient drug to produce an action. Between point A and point C is the duration of action.

decreased renal function as a result of decreased renal blood flow, decreased glomerular filtration rate, and decreased tubular secretion. All of these factors can influence pharmacokinetics. Other problems related to the elderly include the increased incidence of disease states requiring treatment with multiple drugs ("polypharmacy"), which increases the potential for drug interactions and increases incidence of side effects.

Neonates, especially those born prematurely, have a low activity of the hepatic microsomal enzyme system. There is also a poorly developed blood-brain barrier, and an immature mechanism for excretion. All of these factors increase the incidence of toxicity. Children may have an increased drug metabolism, related to the general increase in metabolic rate. Teenagers approach the slower rate seen in adults. This principle applies to most drugs metabolized by the hepatic microsomal enzyme system. Most investigational drug testing is now done in young adult men; for this reason, the effective dose, toxicity, and other factors for infants, children, the elderly, or women of any age are poorly known. The importance of drug testing in the target population is, however, gaining acceptance, and we are currently seeing drug testing in these underinvestigated groups.

2. *Gender.* Women are generally of lower body weight than men and have an increased fat/lean ratio. Sex hormones also may influence drug metabolism and actions. The fluctuating hormonal profile of women during the menstrual cycle may have varying effects on drugs. Again, as most investigational drug testing is not done in women, these influences are poorly understood.

3. *Weight.* Weight affects volume of distribution. For this reason, drug dosage in children is frequently given per kilogram body weight. Also, adipose tissue stores fat-soluble drugs. This may account for the decreased effectiveness of certain drugs in the obese.

4. *Genetic variation.* There may be genetic variation in enzymatic metabolism of drugs. Some people exhibit allergies to some drugs. Certain people are hyporeactors, in that the usual dose produces a lower response. Others are considered hyperreactors, when the usual dose produces an exaggerated response.

5. *Tolerance.* **Tolerance** is defined as when the same dose on repeated occasions produces a lower response, or when a dose increase is required to maintain the same response. This may result from altered metabolism of the drug or a change in the physiological response to the drug. There may be cross-tolerance, in that tolerance to a particular drug may be transferred to another drug producing a similar response. This is especially seen in drugs that have a mood depressing or sedative effect. **Tachyphylaxis** is a rapidly developing tolerance, seen after only a few administrations.

6. *Presence of underlying diseases.* Liver and kidney diseases may affect drug metabolism and excretion. Some drugs are administered as a **pro-drug**. The pro-drug itself is inactive, but after metabolism in the liver, the active metabolite is formed. Pro-drugs may show decreased activity in the presence of liver disease. On the other hand, a drug that is inactivated by the liver may show enhanced activity in the presence of liver disease. Drugs that are excreted by the kidney may be affected by decreased renal function. Knowledge of the drug metabolism is important in prescrib-

ing drugs to people with liver or kidney dysfunction. Frequently, within a drug group there are drugs that are metabolized differently. Thus, one drug may be prescribed for those with liver malfunction and another may be more appropriate for those with kidney disease.

7. *Placebo effect.* The **placebo effect** refers to an improvement in medical status unrelated to an action of a drug. In many studies a placebo effect of 30% is seen. This means that 30% of a study's population show medical improvement even when treated with an inactive substitute. The response to a drug can be affected by a person's emotional state. Interaction with health professionals related to treatment may improve the emotional status of the patient sufficient to improve the patient's medical status. We know the emotional state of a person has an effect on the physical state, although at present we clearly do not understand the impact of emotions or the power of the psyche on wellness.

8. *Compliance.* **Compliance** to a therapeutic regimen requires cooperation of the physician prescribing the drug, the patient, and any others involved in the care of the patient. Communication and understanding of the actions of the drug or reasons for its use, dietary and lifestyle restrictions necessary, manifestations of side effects, and restriction on use of over-the-counter drugs, are required for compliance. Poor compliance can result from problems in communication and understanding between any of the involved parties. The presence of side effects intolerable to the patient can affect compliance. If the patient feels worse taking the drug than not taking the drug, then obviously compliance will be decreased. Frequently, this can be remedied by use of an alternative drug. The use of multiple drugs and complicated and/or changing therapeutic regimens tend to cause decreased compliance. In otherwise healthy patients, a complicated regimen may interfere with lifestyle and decrease compliance. Diminished mental capacity of the patient can affect compliance to any schedule.

Drug interactions

Two drugs administered together or close in time may interact to increase or decrease the intended effect of one or more of the drugs, or may interact to cause a different reaction. Sometimes, interactions preclude use of the two drugs concurrently. More frequently, adjustment in dosage or times of administration is necessary for concurrent use. Drug interactions may be caused by direct interactions between two drugs, competition between two drugs for a plasma protein binding site with displacement of one drug by another, or interactions at the receptor. There also may be drug interactions that occur because physiological responses interact. An **additive effect**, or summation, is seen when the combined effect of two drugs on the same process is the sum of the two individual drugs. This can be used to advantage by prescribing—at reduced dosages—two drugs that have the same physiologic effect; at reduced dosage there is reduced toxicity. A **synergistic effect** is seen when the combined effect is more than the sum of the two drugs. An **antagonistic effect** is when the effect of one drug is counteracted by the effect of another. This may result because of competition at the receptor or because of opposing physiological actions.

A complete drug history is especially important in patients who have more than one physician prescribing drugs. Use of over-the-counter drugs must be included in this history, because many over-the-counter drugs can be involved in drug interactions.

LEARNING OBJECTIVES

1. Understand the different processes involved in pharmacokinetics, including absorption, distribution, metabolism, and elimination.
2. Explain pharmacodynamics, including drug-receptor interactions. Understand the concepts involved in receptor site and the mechanism of action. Describe the difference between agonist and antagonist.
3. Describe the difference between potency and efficacy.
4. Explain several mechanisms for drug interactions.
5. Describe the physiologic consequences of aging as related to altered pharmacokinetics.

ADDITIONAL READINGS

1. Gilman AG, Rall TW, Nies AS, et al (eds): *The Pharmacological Basis of Therapeutics,* ed 8. New York, Pergamon Press, 1990.
2. *Physicians' Desk Reference,* ed 45. Oradell, NJ, Medical Economics Co, 1991.
3. Pratt WB, Taylor P (eds): *Principles of Drug Action: The Basis of Pharmacology,* ed 3. New York, Churchill Livingston, 1990.

Chapter 2

Autonomic Nervous System

The autonomic nervous system is composed of branches of cranial and spinal motor nerves that innervate cardiac muscle, smooth muscle surrounding hollow organs (such as gastrointestinal tract, bladder, and blood vessels) and the exocrine glands (such as the salivary, sweat, tracheobronchial, and secretory glands of the gastrointestinal tract). This visceral motor system, although part of the peripheral nervous system, is not considered to be under conscious control, but is regulated from the hypothalamus and the medulla.

The autonomic nervous system has a particular importance in pharmacology because many drugs interact with autonomic receptors, both adrenergic and cholinergic. These interactions may be of a stimulatory (agonist) or inhibitory (antagonist) nature. In addition, the two transmitters of the autonomic nervous system, acetylcholine and norepinephrine, are transmitters in the central nervous system. Drugs that interact with peripheral autonomic receptors may also interact with these central receptors, if the drugs can cross the blood-brain barrier.

PARASYMPATHETIC NERVOUS SYSTEM

The parasympathetic nervous system, or the craniosacral division of the autonomic nervous system, includes motor fibers of cranial nerves 3, 7, 9, and 10, and sacral nerves S2 through S4. This division regulates the housekeeping functions of the body, such as digestion, excretion, temperature regulation, and urinary bladder contraction. Only specific nerves are stimulated at one time. This gives discrete control of body functions. The various actions of the parasympathetic nervous system are listed in Table 2–1.

Anatomically, the parasympathetic nervous system has long preganglionic nerves emerging from the spinal cord, which synapse in ganglia with the short postganglionic nerves. The ganglia are located near or within the innervated organs. Preganglionic nerve fibers release acetylcholine as their neurotransmitter in the gan-

TABLE 2–1.

Actions of the Parasympathetic Nervous System on Target Organs

Organ	Action
Heart	Decreased heart rate
Gastrointestinal tract	Increased muscle tone, amplitude of contraction, peristalsis; enhanced activity of secretory glands. Enhanced motility may be accompanied by nausea, belching, vomiting, intestinal cramps, diarrhea
Glands	Increased activity of lacrimal, tracheobronchial, salivary, digestive, and exocrine sweat gland secretion
Urinary tract	Increased ureteral peristalsis, contraction of detrusor muscle of urinary bladder, increased maximum voluntary voiding pressure, decreased capacity of bladder
Eye	Miosis (pupil constriction) and accommodation

glia. Short postganglionics then travel in the effector organ and release acetylcholine as the neurotransmitter. Nerves that release acetylcholine are referred to as cholinergic nerves.

Parasympathomimetic agents

Acetylcholine itself cannot be used as a drug because of its diffuseness of actions and rapid degradation. There are three locations of acetylcholine action: (1) in the autonomic ganglia; (2) at the parasympathetic nervous system effector sites; and (3) at the neuromuscular junction. Although acetylcholine acts at all three sites, the receptor types are different. The receptor types are referred to as *muscarinic* at the postganglionic junction, *nicotinic I* in the ganglia, and *nicotinic II* at the neuromuscular junction. With different drugs, the receptors can be stimulated differentially. Agents acting at the muscarinic receptor are described here and are listed in Table 2–2. Drugs that have their effect on the nicotinic receptors will be described later in this chapter, under ganglionic blockers (nicotinic I) and in Chapter 17 in the discussion of myasthenia gravis (nicotinic II).

Muscarinic agents

Bethanechol (Urecholine) is an example of a muscarinic drug. It selectively stimulates the urinary and gastrointestinal tracts by increasing ureteral peristalsis and contraction of the detrusor muscle. In the gastrointestinal tract, both peristalsis and glandular secretion are increased. This agent is useful in treating postoperative and post partum urinary retention, gastric atony (lack of muscle tone, or flaccidity), and abdominal distention. It is also used to stimulate contraction of the urinary bladder after spinal injury, if the vesical reflex is intact (neurogenic bladder). Its use can possibly then avoid catheterization, with the attendant possibility of urinary tract infections.

Possible side effects of muscarinic agents result from their actions on other muscarinic receptors, such as increased sweating, asthma attacks, abdominal cramps, and increased salivation. Contraindications to use of muscarinic agents are asthma, because of increased tracheobronchial secretions and bronchoconstriction; decreased cardiac output resulting in coronary insufficiency, because of possible parasympathomimetic effects on heart rate; and peptic ulcer, because of increased gastric acid secretions.

Antimuscarinic agents

The antimuscarinic agents have actions on several target organs that have clinical significance. Blockade of acetylcholine at the muscarinic receptors produces predictable responses. Because of nonselective blockade, however, there is a high incidence of side effects in organ systems other than the therapeutic target organ. Dry mouth or xerostomia, due to decreased salivation, is a common complaint. This affects oral health and quality of life, interfering with chewing, swallowing, perception of taste and speech. Decreased peristalsis of the small and large intestine leads to constipation. Blockade of the parasympathetic action in the heart leads to tachycardia. Sweat glands are innervated by sympathetic cholinergic nerves. Blockade of these receptors decreases sweating. This probably does not cause a problem with temperature regulation except when other risk factors are present, such as a hot environment or vigorous exercise. Blockade of parasympathetic actions in the eye causes pupil dilation and loss of accommodation. These eye changes cause blurred vision and increased sensitivity to light. The pupil dilation has the potential to precipitate acute angle closure glaucoma in susceptible individuals. There are also muscarinic receptors in cortical and subcortical levels of the brain. Antimuscarinic effects relating to the central nervous system are sedation and mental confusion, ranging from slight memory loss and learning problems to delirium. Although these responses are due to blockade of muscarinic receptors only, they are frequently referred to as anticholinergic responses.

In young adults, the order of appearance of antimuscarinic side effects is as follows: decreased sweating, then decreased nasal and oral secretion; followed by in-

---

TABLE 2–2.

Drugs That Affect the Parasympathetic Nervous System

Muscarinic agents
    Bethanechol (Urecholine)
Antimuscarinic agents
    Decrease respiratory secretion
      Atropine
      Scopolamine
    Bronchial dilation
      Ipratropium bromide (Atrovent)
    Antiparkinsonism
      Trihexyphenidyl (Artane)
      Benztropine mesylate (Cogentin)
      Ethopropazine (Parsidol)
      Orphenadrine (Norflex)

---

creased heart rate, pupil dilation, decreased accommodation, decreased urination, decreased gastrointestinal motility and secretion; and lastly, central nervous system effects. This order may not hold true for the elderly. The elderly are more sensitive to central nervous system effects because of decreased central nervous system cholinergic activity associated with aging. Antimuscarinic side effects are particularly troublesome in the elderly. The onset of symptoms may be gradual but may not be attributable to the drug. Many antimuscarinic effects mimic the common bodily deteriorations associated with aging.

The belladonna alkaloids, such as atropine and scopolamine, are found in many over-the-counter cold medications. The most common action at these low doses is inhibition of bronchial and salivary secretions, resulting in dry mouth. Scopolamine is the most effective drug to prevent motion sickness in most people. It is available in a skin patch, applied behind the ear (Transderm Scōp), and the effects last up to 2 to 3 days. Prophylactic treatment is preferable. It is much less effective if administered after nausea and/or vomiting have occurred. Some anticholinergic drugs are used in treatment of respiratory diseases (Chapter 18) and parkinsonism (Chapter 11) and will be discussed in those chapters.

SYMPATHETIC NERVOUS SYSTEM

The thoracolumbar division of the autonomic nervous system includes outflow in the thoracic and lumbar region of the spinal cord (T-1 to L-3). The short preganglionic nerves emerge from the spinal cord and synapse in the ganglia of the paravertebral sympathetic chain or in the outlying ganglia. The neurotransmitter in the sympathetic ganglia is acetylcholine. The longer postganglionics leave the ganglia and terminate in the various organs. The neurotransmitter released from the postganglionic nerves is norepinephrine. Neurons that release norepinephrine are called adrenergic nerves. Also, the adrenal medulla is considered part of the autonomic nervous system. It is ganglion-like in function, with acetylcholine released by preganglionic nerves in the medulla, causing release of epinephrine and norepinephrine from the medulla into the blood stream. Stimulation of the sympathetic nervous system, including the adrenal medulla, produces changes in the body similar to changes observed during fearful or emergency situations—the "flight or fight" response. In general, all sympathetic nerves are activated, and this is referred to as sympathetic outflow.

The response of an organ to sympathetic nervous system stimulation depends on the presence of specific receptors, the number of receptors, and the affinity of the receptors for either epinephrine or norepinephrine. The different adrenergic receptors have been delineated using specific pharmacologic agents. Thus far, basically three types of receptors have been described: alpha, beta-1, and beta-2. In general, norepinephrine bonds to alpha and beta-1 receptors, and epinephrine binds to all three types of receptors. Alpha receptors are also further subdivided into alpha-1 and alpha-2, with alpha-1 receptors being postsynaptic and alpha-2 receptors being presynaptic. For our purposes, we are most interested in alpha-1 receptors. Table

TABLE 2–3

Adrenergic Receptor Stimulation

Alpha receptor stimulation
  Vasoconstriction
  Pupil dilation (mydriasis)
  Intestinal relaxation
Beta-1 stimulation
  Increased heart rate
  Increased ventricular contractility
Beta-2 stimulation
  Intestinal relaxation
  Bronchodilation

2–3 is a list of responses resulting from stimulation of the different receptor types. Pharmacologically, there are drugs that can stimulate or block the different receptors. Drugs that interact with the sympathetic nervous system are listed in Table 2–4.

Alpha adrenergic agents

The most important clinical effect of the alpha adrenergics is vasoconstriction. Norepinephrine (Levophed) is used clinically in treatment of hypotension associated with shock. Other alpha adrenergic agents may be used to act on mucous membranes of the nasal sinuses to promote decongestion. Phenylephrine (Neo-Synephrine, and others), pseudoephedrine (Sudafed, and others), and phenylpropanolamine (Triaminic, and others) are the most frequently used alpha adrenergics. They are common ingredients in over-the-counter drugs for the relief of nasal and sinus congestion. Topical application of phenylephrine is appropriate as an ophthalmic vasoconstrictor and as a mydriatic, to cause pupil dilation for ophthalmologic examination.

Adverse reactions to alpha adrenergic agents result from overstimulation of the sympathetic nervous system, with central nervous system stimulation experienced as headache, restlessness, anxiety, and tremors. Remember, norepinephrine is also a neurotransmitter in the central nervous system. Overstimulation of the cardiovascular system can lead to hypertension and heart palpitations. The alpha adrenergic agents should not be used by known hypertensive patients or by those taking a monoamine oxidase inhibitor, except under the direction of a physician.

Alpha adrenergic blockers

Alpha blockers block the alpha adrenergic actions of norepinephrine and epinephrine and thus cause vasodilation, leading to a decreased blood pressure. Whenever one part of the autonomic nervous system is blocked, the activity in the other division may be increased. With sympathetic nervous system block, one may see parasympathetic nervous system overactivity, such as nasal congestion and increased gastrointestinal activity.

Phenoxybenzamine (Dibenzyline) is used in peripheral vascular conditions of an adrenergic cause such as Raynaud's phenomenon, when other treatments fail. Raynaud's phenomenon is thought to be a hyperactivity of the sympathetic innervation of the vessels in the extremities, leading to extreme vasoconstriction. Also, it may be used in autonomic hyperreflexia of spinal cord injury, above T-6.

Prazosin (Minipress) is used in treatment of hypertension. It reduces tone in resistance and capacitance vessels, decreases venous return, and decreases cardiac output. The use of alpha blockers in treatment of hypertension is more fully discussed in Chapter 4, Antihypertensive Drugs.

Beta adrenergic agents

The most important target organs that contain beta receptors are the bronchioles and the heart. The heart contains beta-1 receptors, while the bronchioles contain beta-2 receptors. Isoproterenol (Isoprel) is the most potent beta adrenergic drug that interacts with both receptor types, producing bronchodilation and stimulation of the heart. This dual action is the main disadvantage of this drug in treating

TABLE 2–4

Drugs That Affect the Sympathetic Nervous System

Alpha adrenergic agents
   Norepinephrine (Levophed)
   Phenylephrine (Neo-Synephrine; others)
   Pseudoephedrine (Sudafed; others)
   Phenylpropanolamine (Triaminic; others)
Alpha adrenergic blockers
   Phenoxybenzamine (Dibenzyline)
   Prazosin (Minipress)
Beta adrenergic agents
   Mixed
      Isoproterenol (Isoprel)
   Beta-2
      Metaproterenol (Alupent)
Beta adrenergic blockers
   Mixed beta receptor blockers
      Propranolol (Inderal)
      Nadolol (Corgard)
      Pindolol (Visken)
      Timolol (Blocadren)
   Beta-1 receptor blockers
      Atenolol (Tenormin)
      Metoprolol (Lopressor)
      Acebutolol (Sectral)
   Beta blockers with intrinsic sympathetic activity
      Acebutolol (Sectral)
      Pindolol (Visken)
   Ganglionic blockers
      Trimethaphan (Arfonad)
      Mecamylamine (Inversine)

bronchoconstriction caused by asthma or allergy, in that there is usually overstimulation of the heart along with the bronchodilator effect.

A specific beta-2 agonist is metaproterenol (Alupent), which is used to treat bronchoconstriction. The use of beta-2 agonists in treatment of respiratory diseases is discussed in Chapter 18, Respiratory Pharmacology.

Adverse effects of the beta agonists may produce central nervous system stimulation resulting in restlessness, tremor, or anxiety, nausea, and vomiting. Stimulation of cardiac beta receptors causes tachycardia and hypertension. These drugs are used with extreme caution in patients with existing heart disease.

Beta adrenergic blockers

Beta adrenergic blockers are used extensively in treatment of hypertension, angina pectoris, and cardiac arrhythmias. They will be discussed in more detail in the chapters on cardiovascular pharmacology (see Section II).

Propranolol (Inderal) is the oldest of the beta blockers and binds to both beta-1 and beta-2 receptors. Atenolol (Tenormin) is a more specific beta-1 blocker. However, the selectivity of beta-1 blockers is not absolute, and nonspecific blockade of the beta-2 receptors may be seen, especially at the higher doses.

Ganglionic blockers

The ganglionic blockers inhibit neurotransmission in the autonomic ganglia and thus block both the sympathetic and the parasympathetic nervous systems. These agents are used only in severe hypertension that has been unresponsive to more conventional therapy. Specifically, these agents have an important use in autonomic hyperreflexia seen in spinal cord patients (T-6 and above). The common stimulus to cause autonomic hyperreflexia is bladder distention.

The effects of ganglionic blockade depend on the predominate tone or basal autonomic activity to the organs. The predominate tone of arterioles is due to the sympathetic system, so blockade causes dilation. The predominate tone to the gastrointestinal tract and the urinary bladder is parasympathetic stimulation, and so blockade causes decreased muscle tone, with constipation and urinary retention.

Trimethaphan (Arfonad) is used for rapid treatment of hypertensive emergencies. It is available in a solution for intravenous administration. Autonomic hyperreflexia of spinal cord injury is such an emergency. Mecamylamine (Inversine) is used for treatment of moderately severe to severe hypertension that has not responded to more traditional treatment.

PHYSICAL THERAPY NOTES

Many drugs have anticholinergic, really antimuscarinic, side effects. Some of these, such as dry mouth, are generally of minor discomfort and can be relieved by chewing gum or sucking on ice. Other antimuscarinic actions are a concern only with certain preexisting conditions. In a person with compromised respiration, the decreased lung secretion and decreased mucociliary transport may contribute to mucus plugging and development of a respiratory infection.

Many antimuscarinic effects, such as dry mouth, constipation, and memory loss, mimic aging. The onset of symptoms may be gradual and attributed to aging rather than associated with drug side effects.

Autonomic hyperreflexia of spinal injury is most commonly caused by bladder distention, although painful skin stimuli can trigger this reflex. This occurs with a spinal injury above the level of sympathetic splanchnic visceral outflow (injury at T-6 and above). The activation of the sympathetic nervous system causes vasoconstriction and an increase in blood pressure. In a person with an intact spinal cord, this would, reflexively through baroreceptor mechanisms, cause a decreased heart rate and vasodilation. With spinal injury above the level of sympathetic outflow, the heart rate will be decreased, but the vasodilation is prevented.

An autonomic dysfunction can occur in diabetics, as part of the diabetic neuropathy. Orthostatic hypotension and frank syncope may occur. These patients are at risk from falls, so they should avoid sudden changes in posture. For a more complete discussion of orthostatic hypotension, see the section "Postural Hypotension" in Chapter 21.

LEARNING OBJECTIVES

1. Know the anatomic divisions of the autonomic nervous system.
2. List the neurotransmitters released in the autonomic nervous system.
3. Describe the major effects of stimulation of the sympathetic and parasympathetic nervous systems.
4. List the common side effects referred to as antimuscarinic or anticholinergic.
5. Differentiate the adrenergic receptor types and their locations.
6. Describe the effects of blockade or inhibition of the different adrenergic receptor types, and of adverse reactions.

ADDITIONAL READINGS

1. Krum H, Howes LG, Brown DJ, et al: Blood pressure variability in tetraplegic patients with autonomic hyperreflexia. *Paraplegia* 1989; 27:284–288.
2. Mathias CJ: Autonomic dysfunction. *Br J Hosp Med* 1987; 38:238–243.
3. McGuire TJ: Autonomic dysreflexia in the spinal cord-injured. *Postgrad Med* 1986; 80 (Aug):81–89.
4. Peters NL: Antimuscarinic side effects of medications in the elderly. *Arch Intern Med* 1989; 149:2414–2420.
5. Salem MR: Therapeutic uses of ganglionic blocking drugs. *Int Anesthesiol Clin* 1978; 16:171–200.

PART II

Cardiovascular Pharmacology

Heart disease is the leading cause of death in developed countries. Some alterable risk factors are quality and quantity of diet, smoking, level of exercise, and, possibly, stress. A person's genetic pool is also a risk factor for development of cardiovascular disease, but, obviously, it is not alterable.

The function of the heart is to pump blood. For effective function of the heart to occur, there must be (1) sufficient functional muscle cells for contraction, (2) adequate blood flow to the heart cells to provide nutrients, and (3) an intact conduction system for coordination of contraction. The mean arterial pressure is the driving force for flow of blood to the rest of the body. Arterial pressure must be maintained within certain limits. If arterial pressure is below normal (hypotension), insufficient flow delivery will result, with nutrient delivery below the metabolic requirements of the tissues (i.e., ischemia). On the other hand, if arterial pressure is above normal limits (hypertension), the increased pressure can cause damage to the various organs.

Pharmacologic treatment of cardiovascular disease can be directed at any of its symptoms: muscle contraction failure, disturbances in the conduction system, and/or correction of blood flow delivery problems.

Chapter 3

Drugs Used in Treatment of Heart Failure

Heart failure is the inability of the cardiac output to meet the metabolic requirements of the body. Cardiac output (C.O. or $\dot{Q}$) is the product of heart rate and stroke volume. Heart rate is mainly controlled by the autonomic nervous system. Sympathetic nervous system activation increases heart rate, while parasympathetic nervous system stimulation decreases heart rate. Stroke volume is determined by (1) preload, (2) inotropic state, and (3) afterload.

Preload relates to the muscle fiber length at the onset of contraction. As in skeletal muscle, the force of cardiac muscle contraction depends on the initial muscle fiber length. The maximum force of contraction is at the optimal overlap of the actin and myosin filaments of the sarcomere, which allows for the greatest area for their interaction. This relationship forms the basis for the Frank-Starling law of the heart. An increase in the initial volume of the ventricle (end diastolic volume), which is related to the initial muscle length, results in an increased force of contraction, to a limit. End diastolic volume is determined, in part, by venous return. Factors that increase venous return, such as the horizontal position, increased venous tone, and atrial contraction, all tend to increase preload.

Ionic calcium is the principal mediator of the inotropic state of the muscle. Inotropic state, or contractility, is defined as the force of contraction, independent of initial muscle length. Sympathetic tone and circulating catecholamines also influence inotropic state through actions relating to the action of calcium. Both norepinephrine and epinephrine increase ventricular contractility.

Afterload is the tension that the muscle is called upon to develop during contraction, and is dependent on aortic pressure, ventricular wall thickness, and ventricular size. Aortic pressure is the product of cardiac output and total peripheral resistance. Or, in other words, cardiac output is the ratio of aortic pressure to total peripheral resistance. As cardiac output decreases with heart failure, aortic pressure can be maintained by an increase in total peripheral resistance.

In the hearts of healthy individuals, preload (end diastolic volume) is the limiting factor of cardiac output, rather than inotropic state or afterload. In heart failure, at any given end diastolic volume, the force developed during systole is diminished. Thus, a greater end diastolic volume is needed to produce a certain stroke volume. With this mismatch between end diastolic volume and force of contraction, stroke volume decreases. This further increases end diastolic volume, which by the Frank-Starling mechanism, causes a greater force of contraction, up to a limit. When ventricular function becomes depressed and the chamber dilates (no preload reserve), afterload becomes increasingly important in determining cardiac performance.

As heart failure progresses, other compensatory mechanisms occur in an attempt to restore tissue perfusion. These include increased sympathetic nervous system stimulation and increased renin, angiotensin, and aldosterone secretion. These hormones lead to increased salt and water retention to increase the circulating blood volume. This increased volume, however, puts an additional stress on the failing heart. The increased sympathetic nervous system stimulation causes an increased heart rate and inotropic state (i.e., contractility), and an increased total peripheral resistance. The sympathetic nervous system also increases venous tone, with an increase in venous return and an increase in end diastolic volume. The increased salt and water retention also will lead to an increase in venous return, with an increase in end diastolic pressure. With an increased left ventricular end diastolic pressure, there will be an increased pulmonary capillary pressure. When pulmonary capillary pressure exceeds a critical value, pulmonary edema will develop. The increased stiffness of the lungs will increase the work of breathing, leading to dyspnea. With increased right ventricular end diastolic pressure, there is the likelihood of peripheral edema.

These influences of hormonal, neural, or structural changes on the arterial bed that can occur as a compensatory response to the decrease in cardiac output, however, can lead to an increase in afterload. The increased afterload may impose a greater workload on the heart and further reduces cardiac output in a compromised heart, while increasing oxygen requirements. There also may be a diastolic dysfunction, with a limitation to ventricular filling. This is worsened by the tachycardia that decreases the duration of the cardiac cycle spent in diastole, when ventricular filling occurs. Symptoms of heart failure occur when compensatory mechanisms are inadequate to maintain cardiac output appropriate for tissue perfusion or are due to the compensatory mechanisms themselves. In those patients with compensated heart failure, acute heart failure can be precipitated by factors that put an extra load on the heart, such as a systemic infection. A schematic drawing showing the various components of heart failure is show in Figure 3–1.

Dyspnea is the most commonly seen symptom in heart failure. Early in the disease, dyspnea is seen only with exertion. Later, with progression of the heart failure, dyspnea is present also at rest. This is due to increased pressures in the pulmonary capillaries, leading to interstitial edema and causing increased work of inspiration. Orthopnea is respiratory distress in the supine patient and is due to increased ve-

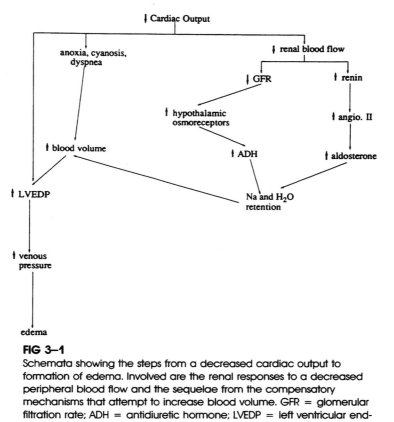

FIG 3–1

Schemata showing the steps from a decreased cardiac output to formation of edema. Involved are the renal responses to a decreased peripheral blood flow and the sequelae from the compensatory mechanisms that attempt to increase blood volume. GFR = glomerular filtration rate; ADH = antidiuretic hormone; LVEDP = left ventricular end-diastolic pressure.

nous return with pooling of blood in the thorax. This may be relieved by pillows under the head and upper thorax. Paroxysmal nocturnal dyspnea is severe shortness of breath that awakens the patient. It is possibly the result of decreased delivery of oxygen to the respiratory center or of decreased sympathetic nervous system activity during sleep and decreased ventricular function.

Unexpected weight gain eventually appears as pitting edema in the lower extremities. This may occur early in heart failure. With advanced heart failure other symptoms from low cardiac output become more evident. With decreased cardiac output there may be decreased cerebral blood flow and symptoms of central nervous system abnormalities. Mental confusion, nausea and vomiting, easy fatigability, chronic tiredness, and insomnia are all related to decreased cerebral perfusion resulting from decreased cardiac output.

Changes in the peripheral vasculature also occur in heart failure. Skeletal muscles no longer function normally. During exercise there is persistent arterial constriction and a decreased oxidative capacity of the muscle. These peripheral changes are the result of more than just reduced blood flow. Immediate improvement of cardiac performance is not associated with immediate enhancement of exercise performance. In fact, improvement in exercise duration may be delayed for up to a few months.

Primary causes of heart failure are the various myopathies (e.g., idiopathic, alcoholic) and connective tissue disorders (e.g., systemic lupus erythematosus). More commonly, heart failure is secondary to other diseases. Atrioventricular valve stenosis causes an obstruction to ventricular filling. Scar tissue formed in response to a myocardial infarction causes loss of ventricular mass and, thereby, loss of function in relation to the size of the infarcted area. Regurgitant atrioventricular valves, atrial septal defects, thyrotoxicosis, and anemia can lead to volume overloads. Hypertension, and obstructions to outflow such as aortic stenosis can lead to pressure overloads. An adaptation to cardiac overload is hypertrophy. However, with hypertrophy there is a contractile disorder in that the increased muscle is inferior, with connective tissue invasion and abnormalities in sarcoplasmic reticulum function and myosin chain structure and function.

Medical management of heart failure includes, in secondary heart failure, treatment of the primary cause, such as hypertension or valvular defects. Restriction of physical activity to allow the heart to rest is indicated. However, complete bed rest may not be warranted for other reasons, such as the chance of phlebothrombosis and pulmonary embolism or the problems associated with the deconditioned state. Also, the recumbent position increases venous return and increases the work of the heart. Emotional rest, with decreased anxiety, is important to reduce sympathetic nervous system activity. A salt-restricted diet is usually recommended. By itself, this may have some benefit. Also, the diuretics, if used, generally have a greater efficacy with a salt-restricted diet. Pharmacologic management of heart failure involves the use of digitalis or other positive inoptropic agent, diuretics, and vasodilators. Treatment regimens using these agents alone or in combination may be attempted in order to best benefit the patient and to minimize risks of drug toxicity.

DRUGS USED IN TREATMENT OF HEART FAILURE

Digitalis

Digitalis, originally found in plants, especially the foxglove, has been used for over 200 years. The two purified digitalis drugs, digitoxin (Crystodigin) and digoxin (Lanoxin), are isolated from different plant species. These are generally similar, but their pharmacokinetics are different. After oral administration, absorption of digoxin is variable—from 40% to 100%, depending on the preparation used. Absorption from tablets depends on their rate and extent of dissolution and may be as low as 40%. Encapsulated digoxin solution (Lanoxicaps) has an absorption rate of almost 100%. Digitoxin absorption from tablets is more complete, almost 100%. Absorption of both is decreased in the presence of food and by malabsorption syndromes. Digoxin is about 25% bound to plasma proteins, while digitoxin is about 95% bound. The elimination half-life of digoxin is about 1½ days, while that for digitoxin is about 7 days. Digoxin is eliminated by renal mechanisms, while hepatic metabolism is the mechanism for digitoxin elimination. In persons with decreased renal blood flow the half-life of digoxin is increased. The onset of action after oral administration is faster for digoxin, from 1½ hours for digoxin, compared to 3 to 6 hours for digitoxin. Digitalis is the term used to refer to all the preparations. The doses needed for initial digitalization and for maintenance therapy depend on the patient's age, body weight, and renal function (for digoxin), and are individually calculated. This is the only class of oral inoptropic agents currently available in the United States. Digoxin is also available for intravenous administration.

In congestive heart failure (muscle failure) there needs to be an increased ability for the heart to contract without increasing oxygen consumption. Digitalis has both direct and indirect actions on the cardiovascular system that are useful in treatment of heart failure. Digitalis directly increases the force of contraction (positive inotropic action) and indirectly, through actions on the autonomic nervous system, slows the heart rate, which allows for increased filling and thus for increased cardiac output. This leads to a decreased heart size, with decreased heart pressures and volumes. Digitalis improves cardiac performance and alleviates symptoms of heart failure by increasing the force of contraction, improving left ventricular function, and increasing cardiac output, and thus increasing tissue perfusion. The action of digitalis to slow ventricular rate makes it useful in treatment of atrial fibrillation or atrial flutter.

The mechanism of action of digitalis is by direct inhibition of the Na^+-K^+-ATPase enzyme in the cell membrane. This decreases active extrusion of sodium, causing an increase in intracellular sodium, which in turn causes an increase in intracellular calcium (decreased Na · Ca exchange). This causes an increase in intracellular stores of calcium, so more calcium is released with each action potential to activate contraction. There is no direct action of digitalis on the contractile elements.

Digitalis also increases parasympathetic nervous system activity and decreases the sensitivity of the heart to sympathetic nervous system activity. Conduction through the atrioventricular node is slowed, which decreases the rate of transmission of atrial impulses to the ventricle. This can lead to a decreased ventricular rate in atrial tachycardia, fibrillation, or flutter, or eventually to atrioventricular node block.

The increased function of the heart and the decreased sympathetic nervous system action then allow for secondary changes. The increased contractility and subsequently increased cardiac output decreases the back pressure through the pulmonary and systemic veins to the capillaries. Pulmonary and peripheral edema are thus relieved. The increased cardiac output, along with the decreased sympathetic activity, maintains arterial pressure with a decreased vascular resistance. This allows for better perfusion of tissues. With improved renal perfusion, the secretion of renin, aldosterone, and antidiuretic hormone are decreased, and the excess fluid is excreted.

Adverse effects
Chronic administration of digitalis is frequently associated with toxicity. The only difference among the different digitalis preparations relates to duration of toxicity.

The preparation with the longer duration of action, digitoxin, leads to a longer duration of toxicity. Overall, digitalis has a low margin of safety. Toxic reactions are frequent, and can be severe or fatal. Children and infants are less sensitive to toxic reactions; however, advanced age increases sensitivity to toxicity because of decreased liver and kidney function and decreased blood flow to these organs. The role of digitalis in treating heart failure is currently undergoing reevaluation because of its toxicity. Traditional medical treatment, with decreased salt intake, decreased activity, and the use of diuretics and vasodilators, may be as effective as digitalis, and result in less toxicity.

The most common cause of toxicity is related to concomitant administration of potassium-depleting diuretics. Patients are likely to develop arrhythmias and conduction abnormalities. However, all disturbances of rhythm are not necessarily the result of digitalis toxicity. Diseased hearts are more likely to develop arrhythmias and conduction disturbances. The increased sensitivity of the heart to digitalis may be due to worsening of the heart failure. Adverse reactions seen are sinus bradycardia, complete atrioventricular block due to enhanced vagal effects, and decreased sympathetic nervous system activity, especially in patients with sinoatrial nodal disease, that is, paroxysmal tachycardia (atria and atrioventricular node). However, paroxysmal tachycardia is also an indication for digitalis treatment. Also seen are ventricular dysrhythmias, such as premature depolarizations, especially coupled (bigeminy and trigeminy); ventricular tachycardia; and ventricular fibrillation. The likelihood and severity of arrhythmias developing from digitalis toxicity are directly related to the severity of the underlying disease, which also increases the likelihood of development of ectopic foci. The antiarrhythmic and proarrhythmic actions of digitalis are complex and are related to the concentration and time of exposure, as well as to the condition of the heart.

Other side effects are nausea, anorexia, vomiting, diarrhea, headache, generalized muscle weakness and easy fatigability, disorientation, confusion, and neuralgic pain in the lower third of the face, simulating trigeminal neuralgia. Nausea and vomiting are also seen in untreated heart failure patients. It is important to differentiate if these symptoms are the result of drug toxicity or worsening of the disease. The side effects may be transitory, entirely absent, or early signs of digitalis intoxication.

Digitalis interacts with other drugs, with the potential for digitalis toxicity. Some of these interactions, other than with the potassium-losing diuretics, are listed in Table 3–1. Phenobarbital, through enhancement of the microsomal enzyme system, increases the metabolism of digitalis. If the digitalis dose is titrated in a patient taking a barbiturate, and the barbiturate is suddenly withdrawn, the digitalis dose will be too high and toxicity will likely develop.

Other inotropic agents

There are other inotropic agents available, or soon to be available. Phosphodiesterase inhibitors, which inhibit the metabolism of adenosine $3':5' =$ cyclic phosphate (cyclic AMP), have been shown to increase myocardial contractility and cause vascular smooth muscle relaxation, leading to peripheral vasodilation. Amrinone

TABLE 3–1

Drug Interactions With Digitalis

Increased metabolism of digitoxin (decreased plasma concentration)
  Barbiturates
  Phenylbutazone (Butazolidin)
  Phenytoin (Dilantin)
Decreased renal excretion of digoxin (increased plasma concentration)
  Quinidine
  Amiodarone (Cordarone)
  Verapamil (Isoptin, Calan)
  Nifedipine (Procardia, Adalat)
  Spironolactone (Aldactone)
  Triamterene (Dyrenium)
  Amiloride (Midamor)
  Nonsteroidal anti-inflammatory agents

(Inocor) (intravenous) and milrinone (Primacor) (oral), are two drugs in this class. Clinical evaluation of their efficacy in treatment of heart failure is ongoing.

Intravenously administered dopamine can act on dopamine, beta-1, and alpha receptors, depending on the dose used. At low doses, stimulation of dopamine receptors in renal, mesenteric, cerebral, and coronary arteries results in dilation of these vascular beds. Increasing blood flow in the renal vascular bed increases the glomerular filtration rate and causes subsequent natriuresis. At moderate doses beta-1 receptors are stimulated causing increased myocardial contractility and cardiac output. Only at high doses does vasoconstriction occur, mediated through the alpha receptors.

Dobutamine (Dobutrex) acts mainly on beta-1 receptors, with actions also on beta-2 and alpha receptors. It has a greater effect on cardiac contractility than on heart rate. Because of its very short half life, about 2 minutes, it must be administered by continuous intravenous infusion. It is useful in short-term treatment of cardiac failure. Although it has a lesser effect on heart rate and blood pressure than other sympathomimetics, it can cause tachycardia and hypertension.

Diuretics

Diuretics are used in heart failure to promote salt and water excretion and reduce plasma volume. The decrease in circulatory volume will lead to decreased left ventricular end diastolic pressure. However, the diuretics do not directly improve ventricular function. Thiazide diuretics are of moderate efficacy and may be used in mild to moderate heart failure, but may not cause sufficient natriuresis in more severe heart failure. Loop diuretics, of greater efficacy, are often preferred in severe heart failure that has been unresponsive to the thiazides and in those patients with frank edema. However, both classes of diuretics cause potassium loss and have the potential to cause hypokalemia, which increases digitalis toxicity. The potassium-

TABLE 3–2

Diuretics

Drug	Total Daily Dose (mg)	Times/Day
High-ceiling diuretics		
Furosemide (Lasix)	20–80	1–2
Ethacrynic acid (Edecrin)	50–200	1–2
Bumetanide (Bumex)	0.5–2	1
Thiazide diuretics		
Chlorothiazide (Diuril)	500–2,000	1–2
Hydrochlorothiazide (Hydrodiuril)	50–200	1–2
Hydroflumethiazide (Diucardin)	25–200	1–2
Bendroflumethiazide (Naturetin)	2.5–5	1
Benzthiazide (Exna)	50–200	1–2
Trichlormethiazide (Metahydrin)	2–4	1–2
Methyclothiazide (Enduron, Aquatensen)	2.5–10	1
Polythiazide (Renese)	1–4	1

sparing agents may be used in combination with the potassium-losing diuretics, allowing a lower dose of each to effect the same degree of natriuresis with fewer side effects. Table 3–2 lists the diuretics and doses used in treatment of heart failure. A more complete discussion of the diuretics is found in Chapter 4, Antihypertensive Drugs.

Vasodilators

Direct acting vasodilators that cause relaxation of arteriolar smooth muscle may be used to relax constricted arterioles. The arteriolar relaxation decreases afterload and may reduce the workload of the heart. These actions may increase tissue perfusion and decrease some compensatory mechanisms seen in heart failure. The direct acting vasodilators are listed in Table 3–3. For a more complete discussion of these drugs see Chapter 4, Antihypertensive Drugs.

Angiotensin Converting Enzyme Inhibitors

Angiotensin converting enzyme (ACE) inhibitors may be effective in mild to moderate heart failure. The ACE inhibitors inhibit conversion of angiotensin I to

TABLE 3–3

Vasodilators

Drug	Total Daily Dose (mg)	Times/Day
Hydralazine (Apresoline)	40–200	4
Minoxidil (Loniten)	5–40	1–2

angiotensin II. Angiotensin II is a potent vasoconstrictor. By preventing the formation of angiotensin II these drugs decrease arteriolar and venous constriction, thus reducing afterload and preload, and breaking the vicious cycle of heart failure. Some deleterious effects of the compensatory mechanisms in heart failure seem to be due to an increased activity of the angiotensin-renin system. Inhibition of this system may allow for improvement in salt and water homeostasis. Table 3–4 is a list of the ACE inhibitors and doses used in treatment of heart failure. See Chapter 4, Antihypertensive Drugs, for a more complete discussion of the various drugs.

PHYSICAL THERAPY NOTES

Bed rest is indicated for acute, unstable heart failure. However, in medically stable patients, an exercise program is necessary as part of the total management of the patient. Prevention of some disabling effects of deconditioning can be aided by just the upright position. The upright position also favorably affects fluid compartments. Conditioning needs to progress with consideration for the patient's overall clinical situation. Shortness of breath adds to the patient's anxiety and increases sympathetic nervous system stimulation, which increases the work of the heart. Thus, there is a delicate and individual balance between not making the situation worse and improving the overall clinical outlook for the patient.

Muscular weakness and easy fatigability are associated with both worsening of heart failure and with digitalis toxicity.

LEARNING OBJECTIVES

1. Understand the progression of heart failure and the physiologic compensations made to adjust for the decrease in stroke volume that maintain tissue perfusion.
2. List the primary causes of heart failure.
3. Describe the different classes of drugs used to treat heart failure and their mechanisms.
4. Explain the toxicity of digitalis, especially related to plasma potassium concentration.

TABLE 3–4

Angiotensin Converting Enzyme Inhibitors

Drug	Total Daily Dose (mg)	Times/Day
Captopril (Capoten)	150–300	3
Enalapril (Vasotec)	5–20	2
Lisinopril (Zestril, Prinivil)	20–40	1

ADDITIONAL READINGS

1. Brozena S, Jessup M: Pathophysiologic strategies in the management of congestive heart failure. *Annu Rev Med* 1990; 41:65–74.
2. Geltman EM: Mild heart failure: diagnosis and treatment. *Am Heart J* 1989; 118:1277–1291.
3. Katz AM: Cardiomyopathy of overload. *N Engl J Med* 1990; 322:100–110.
4. Mancini DM, LeJemtel TH, Factor S, et al: Central and peripheral components of cardiac failure. *Am J Med* 1986; 80 (suppl 2B):2–13.
5. Manmontri A, MacLeod SM: Centrally acting sympatholytic agents in the treatment of congestive heart failure. *Drugs* 1990; 40:169–175.
6. Smith TW: Digitalis. *N Engl J Med* 1988; 318:358–365.
7. Sonnenblick EH, LeJemtel TH: Pathophysiology of congestive heart failure. *Am J Med* 1989; 87 (suppl 6B):88S–91S.

Chapter 4

Antihypertensive Drugs

Mean arterial blood pressure is the driving force of blood flow to the organs. Long-term maintenance of arterial blood pressure within normal limits is due partly to hormonal mechanisms and partly to renal mechanisms. The major hormonal control of long-term blood pressure maintenance is the renin-angiotensin system. Renin is an enzyme secreted from the kidney that causes the conversion of angiotensinogen to angiotensin I. Angiotensinogen is a protein secreted from the liver that circulates in the blood. The activation of angiotensin I to angiotensin II is due to converting enzyme which is located on the inner surface of capillaries. Angiotensin II is a very potent vasoconstrictor and it also stimulates the adrenal cortex to secrete aldosterone. Aldosterone is a hormone that acts in the distal tubule to increase sodium reabsorption and potassium secretion. In conditions of decreased blood perfusion of the kidney, renin is released. Renin, through an increase in angiotensin II, stimulates vasoconstriction in an attempt to increase blood pressure, and thus restore renal perfusion. The increased aldosterone secretion causes an increase in renal sodium reabsorption, which is followed by water reabsorption. This leads to an increase in extracellular fluid volume, as an attempt to increase blood pressure. Conversely, if pressure is too high, renin secretion will be inhibited.

Normal kidney function is also required for long-term maintenance of blood pressure. The kidney output of salt and water is related to arterial pressure. In other words, as arterial pressure rises, the kidney output of salt and water will increase in order to decrease extracellular fluid volume and thus return blood pressure to normal limits.

Hypertension, generally characterized by higher than normal arterial systolic and diastolic blood pressures (greater than 140/90 mmHg), is a leading cause of cerebral strokes, heart attacks, and kidney disease. Hypertension is classified as mild (150/90), moderate (180/100), or severe (greater than 210/115). In the elderly, systolic hypertension may occur, and is defined as a systolic blood pressure greater than 160 mm Hg.

In about 10% of hypertensive patients the hypertension is secondary to another disease, such as a tumor of the adrenal medulla (pheochromocytoma), hypercortisolism (Cushing's syndrome), or renal disease. This latter should be distinguished from renal damage caused by hypertension. In the other 90% of hypertensive patients, the causative factor is not known; this primary, or essential, hypertension, is probably due to some disturbance in the long-term control of blood pressure. Hypertension is not thought to result from a lack of control of the baroreceptor reflex, which is a short-term blood pressure control mechanism.

Although the cause is not known, primary, or essential, hypertension is associated with certain risk factors. These include race, family history of hypertension, obesity, cigarette smoking, hyperglycemia, hypercholesterolemia, preexisting cardiovascular disease (angina or heart failure), and a history of a previous stroke. Nonpharmacologic treatment should be attempted in all patients. Nonpharmacologic adjustments include dietary reduction of sodium intake, weight loss if the person is obese, moderation of alcohol intake, cessation of smoking, increased exercise, and reduction of stress. These nonpharmacologic changes may be sufficient treatment in those with mild hypertension, and they also enhance the antihypertensive actions of most of the drugs.

Pharmacologic reduction of blood cholesterol levels, if elevated, and control of diabetes mellitus are also included in treatment of hypertension. Because the cause of most cases of hypertension is not known, the goal of drug therapy is aimed at lowering blood pressure and not at the cause of hypertension. This goal must include not producing excessive adverse effects to the patient. Antihypertensive drug therapy should not aggravate known heart disease risk factors, such as hyperlipidemia. In order to prolong a useful life by preventing cardiovascular complications, treatment schedules should interfere as little as possible with the patient's acceptable lifestyle. Since this is a lifelong treatment, and may require a change in lifestyle, compliance may be a problem. In those people with asymptomatic mild hypertension, acceptance of side effects is variable. Does treatment of hypertension really prolong life, or just make it seem longer? All antihypertensive agents have the potential to cause impotence in men. Some classes of drugs are more likely than others, and men have different susceptibility to this side effect from different drugs.

Simple treatment schedules improve compliance to chronic drug treatment. The first four groups to be discussed (diuretics, beta blockers, calcium channel blockers, and angiotensin converting enzyme inhibitors) have been successfully used as monotherapy. The others (central alpha agonists, peripheral alpha antagonists, and direct acting vasodilators) generally require addition of a second agent because although they do reduce blood pressure, physiologic compensation to the reduction in pressure negates the antihypertensive effect.

DIURETICS

Diuretics have been the mainstay of treatment of hypertension for many years. Initially, these agents cause an intravascular volume contraction with a subsequent decrease in cardiac output. After several weeks of treatment, the plasma volume

TABLE 4-1.

Thiazide Diuretics

Drug	Total Daily Dose (mg)	Times/Day
Chlorothiazide (Diuril)	500–1,000	1–2
Hydrochlorothiazide (Hydrodiuril)	50–100	1–2
Hydroflumethiazide (Diucardin)	50–100	1–2
Bendroflumethiazide (Naturetin)	2.5–15	1
Benzthiazide (Exna)	50–200	2
Trichlormethiazide (Metahydrin)	2–4	1–2
Methyclothiazide (Enduron, Aquatensen)	2.5–5	1
Polythiazide (Renese)	2–4	1

and cardiac output return to pretreatment levels, but the total peripheral resistance decreases. The decrease in total peripheral resistance seems to be the long-term mechanism of blood pressure reduction. These drugs may be used alone, or in combination with a drug from another class.

Concurrent administration of nonsteroidal anti-inflammatory drugs (NSAIDs), such as aspirin, with diuretics reduces the efficacy of diuretics and may cause salt and water retention. This is due to inhibition of prostaglandin synthesis by the NSAIDs and demonstrates the importance of prostaglandins in normal renal function. Diuretics can increase the toxicity of lithium, an antipsychotic drug used in treating manic episodes, which warrants adjustment of the lithium dose. The bile acid binding resins used to treat hypercholesterolemia may impair absorption of certain drugs if used simultaneously.

Thiazide Diuretics

Thiazide diuretics inhibit sodium reabsorption in the early distal tubule, causing an increased secretion of potassium and a resultant loss of sodium, potassium, chloride, and water in the urine. The thiazide diuretics are listed in Table 4-1. Chlorothiazide (Diuril), the prototype of this group, has an onset of action in about 1 to 2 hours and a duration of action of 6 to 12 hours. It is eliminated by the kidney as the intact molecule. Because of the importance of the kidney in its elimination, this drug should be used with caution in those patients with renal disease.

Thiazides may be the drug of choice in mild to moderate hypertension and heart failure. The thiazides are more likely to be effective in the elderly and in blacks, who generally have low-renin hypertension. However, the elderly may be prone to orthostatic hypotension and syncope if they are previously volume contracted. These agents are more effective as antihypertensives than the high-ceiling, or nonthiazide, diuretics in patients without edema. Several weeks of therapy with the thiazide may be required before optimal clinical responses are evident.

Potassium loss is frequently related to the dose of the thiazide diuretic, but frank

TABLE 4-2.

High-Ceiling Diuretics

Drug	Total Daily Dose (mg)	Times/Day
Furosemide (Lasix)	80	1–2
Ethacrynic acid (Edecrin)	50–200	1-2
Bumetanide (Bumex)	0.5–2	1

hypokalemia may occur at any dose. Hypokalemia may increase the toxicity of digitalis, which is used in treatment of heart failure. A sodium-restricted diet may minimize this potassium loss. A reduction in dietary salt intake allows for lower doses of the thiazide to be used, thus reducing the risk of side effects. Thiazides also have the potential for producing hyperglycemia and hypercholesterolemia. For this reason, they may not be suitable for patients with diabetes mellitus and other metabolic disorders. Hyperuricemia may develop from thiazide treatment, with precipitation of gout. The thiazides may cause fatigue in some patients and impotence in men. In spite of this, low-dose therapy with thiazide diuretics is well tolerated and generally without side effects.

Hypokalemia symptoms are muscle weakness, fatigue, cardiac arrhythmias, and potentiation of digitalis toxicity. Thiazide diuretics may be used in combination with a potassium-sparing diuretic to obtain an additive diuretic effect and still maintain potassium balance, or with potassium supplements. Diuretic effects are additive between classes of diuretics, but not within classes.

High-Ceiling or Loop Diuretics

The high-ceiling diuretics have a higher efficacy on volume excretion than the thiazides. They inhibit sodium chloride transport in the ascending limb of the loop of Henle, with increased secretion of potassium in the distal tubule because of the increased sodium load delivered to the distal tubule. The high-ceiling diuretics have short half-lives, with durations of action of about 3 to 6 hours, and are mainly excreted by the kidney. Drugs classified as high-ceiling or loop diuretics are listed in Table 4-2. Only furosemide (Lasix) is approved for treatment of hypertension. All are approved for treatment of edema resulting from heart failure.

Furosemide is used to treat acute pulmonary edema or hypertension that is resistant to other diuretics. Hypokalemia can result, which is generally dose related. Furosemide is more toxic than the thiazides, but is more likely to be effective in those individuals with frank edema.

Abnormalities of fluid and electrolyte imbalance are the most common forms of toxicity. The increased secretion of titratable acid and ammonia is the cause for diuretic-induced metabolic alkalosis. Binding to plasma proteins and competition for binding sites account for adverse drug interactions, especially with warfarin (Coumadin), an anticoagulant, and clofibrate (Atromid-S), a lipid-lowering drug.

TABLE 4–3.

Potassium-Sparing Diuretics

Drug	Total Daily Dose (mg)	Times/Day
Spironolactone (Aldactone)	50–100	1–2
Triamterene (Dyrenium)	200	2
Amiloride (Midamor)	5–10	1

Potassium-Sparing Diuretics

Spironolactone (Aldactone) is a competitive antagonist to aldosterone action, and thus inhibits sodium reabsorption and potassium secretion in the distal tubule. Triamterene (Dyrenium) and amiloride (Midamor), although they are not aldosterone antagonists, resemble spironolactone in that they are potassium sparing. The potassium-sparing diuretics are listed in Table 4–3. Spironolactone and triamterene are mainly metabolized by the liver. Amiloride is not metabolized, but is excreted unchanged by the kidney.

These drugs do not cause potassium loss; however, potassium retention may occur, with hyperkalemia developing. They may be used in combination with potassium-losing diuretics, as mentioned earlier. The combination allows for a lower dose of each to be used to attain the same result, with fewer side effects.

BETA BLOCKERS

Beta blockers are the second most popular class of drugs used in treatment of hypertension. They block the actions of endogenous epinephrine and norepinephrine on beta receptors and thus inhibit renin release and reduce cardiac output by decreasing heart rate and cardiac contractility, all through a beta-1 effect. Mixed beta blockers also block beta-2 receptors in the bronchioles and can cause respiratory distress in susceptible individuals. Beta blockers with intrinsic sympathetic activity, the so-called partial agonists, may have an advantage in that they decrease total peripheral resistance without changing resting heart rate or cardiac output. Beta blockers are more effective in younger patients, or in those with high renin levels. The beta blockers are listed in Table 4–4.

Propranolol (Inderal) is the oldest of the beta blockers and blocks both beta-1 and beta-2 receptors. Atenolol (Tenormin) is a more specific beta-1 blocker; however, the selectivity of beta-1 blockers is not absolute. The beneficial results of beta blockade are a lowering of blood pressure and a decrease in the work of the cardiovascular system. Beta blockers are effective treatment for those patients with coexisting coronary artery disease, with angina and supraventricular arrhythmias.

Propranolol is metabolized by the liver. However, there is a lot of individual variation in metabolism and, thus, in plasma concentration. Fine-tune dosing can be achieved by clinical measurement of heart rate and blood pressure. Dosing once or

TABLE 4–4.

Beta Blockers

Drug	Total Daily Dose (mg)	Times/Day
Mixed beta blockers		
Propranolol (Inderal)	120–240	2–3
Nadolol (Corgard)	40–80	1
Pindolol (Visken)	10–60	2
Timolol (Blocadren)	20–40	2
Beta-1 blockers		
Atenolol (Tenormin)	50–100	1
Metoprolol (Lopressor)	100–450	2
Acebutolol (Sectral)	400–800	2
Intrinsic sympathetic activity		
Acebutolol (Sectral)	400–800	2
Pindolol (Visken)	10–60	2

twice daily may be sufficient for the antihypertensive effect. There is a sustained-release preparation (Inderal LA) that may improve patient compliance.

Beta blockers, however, should not be used when heart function is excessively reduced, that is, when the ejection fraction is less than 40%. Blockade of beta-1 receptors usually produces bradycardia and may lead to congestive heart failure or cardiac arrest in an already compromised heart. These problems can generally be avoided by careful patient selection. A person on a beta blocker does not show normal cardiovascular responses to exercise. The increases in heart rate and contractility mediated through the beta receptors are blocked. The Frank-Starling law is still in effect, so cardiac output increase is dependent on venous return. There are some beta receptor independent increases in heart rate. Overall, the cardiovascular response to exercise in patients taking beta blockers is more variable. Beta blockers, except those with intrinsic sympathetic activity, increase plasma triglycerides and decrease high density lipoprotein-cholesterol levels. Diabetics on beta blockers do not experience normal responses to hypoglycemia. Beta blockers inhibit the epinephrine counterregulatory actions and the increased heart rate in response to hypoglycemia. For these reasons, other antihypertensive agents are more appropriate for diabetic patients. Propranolol should be used with extreme caution in patients with respiratory conditions. Otherwise, the beta blockers are generally well tolerated.

The most frequently reported side effects to beta blockers are muscular weakness, decreased exercise tolerance, and cold extremities. Nausea, vomiting, diarrhea, and constipation have also been reported. Central nervous system actions may produce depression, hallucinations, nightmares, insomnia, and dizziness. Sudden withdrawal of beta blockers may cause a life-threatening syndrome characterized by ventricular arrhythmias, severe angina, myocardial infarction, and even death (rebound hypersensitivity). Gradual discontinuance of a beta antagonist over a period of 7 to 14 days has been recommended to prevent these severe withdrawal reactions.

TABLE 4–5.

Indications for Calcium Channel Blockers

Drug	Arrhythmias	Angina Pectoris		Hypertension
		Spasm	Stable	
Diltiazem		+	+	
Nicardipine			+	+
Nifedipine		+	+	
Verapamil	+	+	+	+
Isradipine				+

* + = approved indication.

CALCIUM CHANNEL BLOCKERS

The calcium channel blockers inhibit the slow calcium channels in cardiac and smooth muscle cells. They thus inhibit entry of calcium into cells or inhibit its mobilization from intracellular stores. The calcium channel blockers are direct arterial dilators with little effect on the venous beds. They cause dilation of coronary arteries, with a reduction in coronary vascular resistance. They also accelerate relaxation of ventricles, and improve subendocardial perfusion. The direct negative inotropic and chronotropic effects of the calcium channel blockers limit reflex sympathetic activation of myocardial function, which normally occurs as peripheral resistance falls. These drugs are also likely to disturb atrioventricular conduction. In individuals without heart failure, ventricular performance is unimpaired; however, in persons with heart failure, drug use may lead to decreased contractility and decreased left ventricular function. The calcium channel blockers are generally more effective in those patients with low-renin hypertension (e.g., the elderly and blacks). Some of these agents are also effective treatment for coronary artery disease with angina, variant (Prinzmetal's) angina, and certain arrhythmias, so they may be advantageously used in patients with these diseases in addition to hypertension. The calcium channel blockers and indications for their use are listed in Table 4–5.

These agents are well absorbed after oral administration and are extensively protein bound. They are metabolized in the liver. Because of their relatively short half-lives, each drug must be administered 3 or 4 times per day. Verapamil (Isoptin) is available in a long-acting formulation (Isoptin Sustained Release). In the elderly with decreased liver metabolism, the elimination half-life may be extended. If dosage and/or times of administration are not adjusted, the plasma concentration may increase and increase the incidence of side effects.

There are currently five calcium channel blockers approved for treatment of cardiovascular diseases (hypertension, angina, and arrhythmias). The three approved for treatment of hypertension are verapamil (Isoptin, Calan) nicardipine (Cardene), and isradipine (DynaCirc) (Table 4–6). Verapamil and nicardipine have been used for several years, so more is known about their side effects. Isradipine was released in the United States in 1990, so the data on long-term administration are less clear.

TABLE 4–6.

Calcium Channel Blockers

Drug	Total Daily Dose (mg)	Times/Day
Verapamil (Isoptin, Calan)	240–360	3
Nicardipine (Cardene)	60–120	3
Isradipine (DynaCirc)	2.5–5.0	2

The most frequently observed side effect of verapamil (Isoptin, Calan) is constipation, which may be treated with a stool softener. Verapamil alters heart rate conduction and should not be used in those patients with sinus node disease or second or third degree atrioventricular block. Nicardipine (Cardene) can cause excessive vasodilation and associated reflex stimulation of the sympathetic nervous system, with headache, tachycardia, flushing, and pedal edema occurring. Nicardipine is also reported to increase the frequency, duration, and severity of angina. Isradipine (DynaCirc) is reported to have fewer undesirable effects on heart function. All the calcium channel blockers are contraindicated in severe heart failure, hypotension, or in cases of increased angina. The calcium blockers reportedly have no effect on plasma lipid profiles.

ANGIOTENSIN CONVERTING ENZYME INHIBITORS

The angiotensin converting enzyme (ACE) inhibitors inhibit conversion of angiotensin I to angiotensin II. Angiotensin II is a potent vasoconstrictor and a stimulus for aldosterone secretion by the adrenal cortex. Aldosterone causes an increase in distal tubule sodium reabsorption. Both the vasoconstriction and the increased sodium retention can be associated with hypertension. The ACE inhibitors lower systemic arteriolar resistance, and mean, diastolic, and systolic pressures, without increasing heart rate, cardiac output, or contractility. Both preload and afterload are decreased. Arteriolar dilation reduces afterload, and the decreased excess volume causes decreased preload. Blood flow in the coronary and cerebral beds is maintained by autoregulation, and baroreceptor function and cardiac reflexes are not altered. The ACE inhibitors are listed in Table 4–7.

The drugs in this class of antihypertensive agents are generally well tolerated, especially if used with a diuretic. The gastrointestinal absorption of captopril (Capoten) is decreased by the presence of food, so it should be taken at least 1 hour before meals. Although it has a half-life of 2 hours, its effects last longer and it can be given two or three times a day. Most of the drug is excreted by the kidney. Thus, plasma concentration can be increased in the presence of impaired renal function.

The ACE inhibitors may be used in mild to moderate hypertension. They have no sympathetic blocking activity, so postural hypotension is rare, and the cardiovas-

TABLE 4–7.

Angiotensin Converting Enzyme Inhibitors

Drug	Total Daily Dose (mg)	Times/Day
Captopril (Capoten)	50–450	2–3
Enalapril (Vasotec)	10–40	1–2
Lisinopril (Zestril, Prinivil)	20–40	1

cular response to exercise is normal. These agents are effective in patients with normal or elevated renin levels. They do not alter the plasma lipid profile so they may be more appropriate in those patients with hyperlipidemia. As mentioned earlier, these drugs should be used with caution in patients with impaired renal function. On the positive side, the ACE inhibitors rarely cause impotence. Tolerance to the antihypertensive action does not develop, so abrupt withdrawal of these agents is not associated with rebound hypertension.

Captopril (Capoten), enalapril (Vasotec), and lisinoprin (Zestril, Prinivil) are the three ACE inhibitors approved for use in the United States. Side effects, more likely with captopril than with the others, include hypotension, hyperkalemia, cough, and renal failure. Cough, a fairly common side effect, is usually nocturnal and is of a nonproductive nature. Hyperkalemia is usually not a problem in those patients with normal renal function. The risk of hyperkalemia is increased with the concomitant use of potassium-sparing diuretics, potassium supplements, NSAIDs, and in those patients with impairment of renal function and diabetes mellitus. Transient side effects are mainly gastrointestinal, and may disappear with continued treatment. These drugs interact with the NSAIDs, which may increase the risk of hyperkalemia in those taking ACE inhibitors. Also, the NSAIDs can negate the antihypertensive actions of ACE inhibitors.

CENTRAL ACTING ALPHA AGONISTS

The centrally acting alpha agonists are the third most popular drug class used in treatment of hypertension. These drugs are listed in Table 4–8. They act to decrease central sympathetic outflow, thus decreasing arterial pressure, which is not accompanied by reflex tachycardia. With long-term treatment, there is a decrease in total peripheral resistance. Cardiac output and myocardial oxygen consumption in response to exercise remain unchanged from pretreatment levels.

Methyldopa (Aldomet) is rapidly absorbed after oral administration, but its effects are not seen for 6 to 8 hours after administration; probably because it is transported into the central nervous system where it exerts its action. Although methyldopa has a short plasma half-life, its plasma concentration has no relation to its action, again because its site of action is in the central nervous system. It is excreted by the kidneys and is generally administered once or twice a day. Clonidine

TABLE 4–8.

Central Acting Alpha Agonists

Drug	Total Daily Dose (mg)	Times/Day
Methyldopa (Aldomet)	500–2,000	2–4
Clonidine (Catapres)	0.2–0.6	2
Guanabenz (Wytensin)	8–64	2

(Catapres) is available in tablet form and also in a transdermal patch, which requires changing only once a week. The only problem with this formulation may be contact dermatitis.

The centrally acting alpha agonists decrease total peripheral resistance, especially arterial pressure, without much change in cardiac output or heart rate in younger patients. In older patients, however, they may cause venous relaxation, thus a reduction in preload, which leads to a decrease in stroke volume and cardiac output. Orthostatic hypotension is generally less severe than with drugs that act on the peripheral autonomic nervous system. These drugs do not block the baroreceptor reflex. Side effects are drowsiness and decreased mental alertness, dry mouth, impotence, dizziness, and enhanced hypotension. These drugs are generally used with a diuretic to prevent fluid retention. Rapid withdrawal can cause a hypertensive crisis, and—similar to the beta blockers—withdrawal should be gradual, over 7 to 14 days.

PERIPHERAL ALPHA ANTAGONISTS

The peripheral alpha antagonists block the actions of epinephrine and norepinephrine on the alpha receptors in the arterioles and veins. Thus, they reduce tone in both resistance and capacitance vessels. This then decreases venous return and decreases cardiac output. Thus, there is a decrease in both preload and afterload. Prazosin (Minipress) causes little reflex tachycardia; however, this may occur on standing as a result of hypotension. It is best used with a beta blocker or a diuretic. Orthostatic hypotension and syncope may occur early in treatment, but tolerance generally develops with long-term use. Prazosin improves the lipoprotein profile, so it may have an advantage in those patients with metabolic disorders. The cerebral and coronary beds are not affected. Cardiovascular response to exercise is not affected. The peripheral alpha antagonists are listed in Table 4–9.

Prazosin is well absorbed after oral administration and is highly bound to plasma proteins. Decreases in plasma proteins, as may occur with some diseases, lead to an increase in the amount of free drug. It has a duration of action of 4 to 6 hours, and must be administered two or three times per day.

TABLE 4–9.

Peripheral Alpha Blockers

Drug	Total Daily Dose (mg)	Times/Day
Prazosin (Minipress)	6–15	2–3
Terazosin (Hytrin)	1–5	1

DIRECT ACTING VASODILATORS

The direct acting vasodilators decrease total peripheral resistance by relaxation of arteriolar smooth muscle. Hydralazine (Apresoline; Table 4–10) decreases diastolic pressure more than systolic pressure because of dilation of arterioles rather than veins, so postural hypotension is rare. It may, however, cause a reflex increase in sympathetic nervous system activity, with increased heart rate and contractility. It also increases renin secretion and may cause water retention. Because of these actions on salt and water homeostasis, drugs in this class are best used in combination with a diuretic. The directing acting vasodilators do not affect blood lipids or glucose. Minoxidil (Loniten) is similar to hydralazine, but has the unique side effect of hypertrichosis, which may limit or add to its usefulness. Minoxidil is the active ingredient in Rogaine, which is used topically to stimulate hair growth.

The metabolism of hydralazine is fairly unique in that a genetically determined metabolism of the drug occurs in the gastrointestinal tract. Fifty percent of the population rapidly metabolize this drug, so a higher dose is needed to produce the same response. This difference in metabolism occurs before the drug reaches the plasma, so plasma half-life is not affected. Plasma half-life is about 1 hour, but the duration of action is 12 hours.

PHYSICAL THERAPY NOTES

In monitoring of heart rate response to exercise, note whether the antihypertensive drug affects exercise response. Beta blockers, as a rule, do blunt the heart rate response to exercise.

Orthostatic hypotension may be a problem with some patients on antihypertensives. The elderly generally are more susceptible to this side effect. Peripheral alpha antagonists may cause orthostatic hypotension, especially early in treatment. Tolerance to this generally develops. Central alpha agonists also may cause hypotension, but generally less frequently than the peripherally acting agents. Diuretics may cause postural hypotension, if the patient is volume contracted. The direct acting vasodilators rarely cause hypotension if the baroreceptor reflex is intact. Importantly, the sensitivity of the baroreceptor reflex tends to decrease with aging. Also, diabetics may have an autonomic neuropathy, which interferes with the baroreceptor reflex.

TABLE 4–10

Direct Acting Vasodilators

Drug	Total Daily Dose (mg)	Times/Day
Hydralazine (Apresoline)	40–200	4
Minoxidil (Loniten)	5–40	1

The ACE inhibitors and the calcium channel blockers rarely cause orthostatic hypotension.

Postural hypotension resulting from a delayed baroreceptor response may occur in the elderly, especially in the presence of a drug capable of producing hypotension. Susceptible individuals are at risk for injuries resulting from falls. Moving the feet and legs, while in the sitting position, with active dorsiflexion, may stimulate sufficient venous return to prevent a serious drop in blood pressure upon standing. The patient needs to be instructed to arise slowly to a sitting position, and then to standing. For more information on postural hypotension, see Chapter 21.

Blacks and the elderly are more likely to have low-renin hypertension and generally respond better to diuretics than to beta blockers or ACE inhibitors. The younger population of caucasians is more likely to have normal or high renin hypertension and respond to beta blockers or ACE inhibitors. The other classes of drugs are the same in both races.

LEARNING OBJECTIVES

1. Understand the basic physiology of blood pressure control, both short-term and long-term mechanisms.
2. Explain the basic groups of diuretics and the different sites of action within the kidney.
3. Know which diuretics cause potassium loss and the specific symptoms associated with hypokalemia.
4. Know the classes of drugs used to treat hypertension and the antihypertensive actions of these drugs (i.e., diuretics, beta blockers, calcium channel blockers, ACE inhibitors, central alpha agonists, peripheral alpha antagonists, and direct acting vasodilators).
5. From an understanding of the mechanisms of action of the antihypertensive drugs, describe the combinations of drugs that may be used and why the combinations are effective.

ADDITIONAL READINGS

1. 1988 Joint National Committee: The 1988 report of the joint national committee on de-

tection, evaluation, and treatment of high blood pressure. *Arch Intern Med* 1988; 148:1023–1038.

2. Andren L: General considerations in selecting antihypertensive agents in patients with type II diabetes mellitus and hypertension. *Am J Med* 1989; 87(suppl 6A):39S–41S.

3. Braunwald E: Mechanism of action of calcium-channel-blocking agents. *N Engl J Med* 1982; 307:1618–1627.

4. Dzau VJ; Atherosclerosis and hypertension: Mechanisms and interrelationships. *J Cardiovasc Pharmacol* 1990; 15(suppl 5):S59–S64.

5. Ferrario CM: The renin-angiotensin system: Importance in physiology and pathology. *J Cardiovasc Pharmacol* 1990; 15(suppl 3):S1–S5.

6. Messerli FH, Kaesser UR, Losem CJ: Effects of antihypertensive therapy on hypertensive heart disease. *Circulation* 1989; 80(suppl IV):IV-145–IV-150.

7. Rahn KH: Principles of antihypertensive drug treatment. *Am J Cardiol* 1990; 65:82G–84G.

8. Schoenberger JA: Controversies in the use of combination therapy in the older patient. *Drugs* 1990; 39(suppl 2):64–66.

Chapter 5

Antiarrhythmic Drugs

The conducting system of the heart consists of specialized cardiac muscle cells containing few contractile fibrils. These cells exhibit automaticity. That is, in these cells, the resting potential spontaneously depolarizes to threshold, generating another action potential. The sinoatrial node is the normal pacemaker of the heart because it has the highest automatic rate. This rate, however, can be influenced by the autonomic nervous system. Stimulation of the sympathetic nervous system increases the rate of spontaneous depolarization, while stimulation of the parasympathetic system decreases the rate. The action potential exits the sinoatrial node and passes throughout the atria along the intranodal pathways. This causes contraction of the atria. The atrioventricular node delays the passage of the action potential, which allows for contraction of the atria before the ventricles contract. This delay is important in that it allows for ventricular filling. The bundle of His exits from the atrioventricular node and enters the interventricular septum, where it splits into the left and right bundle branches. Branches from these bundles give rise to the Purkinje system, which extends throughout the subendocardium of the ventricles. The rapid conduction of the action potential throughout the ventricles by the Purkinje system allows for simultaneous contraction of the muscle fibers of the ventricles. Pacemaker foci other than the sinoatrial node are considered ectopic and may lead to uncoordinated contraction of atria and ventricles. Arrhythmias can be due to abnormalities in impulse generation and/or in impulse propagation.

The atrioventricular bundle is normally the only pathway for electrical impulses between the atria and the ventricles. The rest of the atrioventricular septum is connective tissue, which does not conduct electrical impulses. Sometimes, however, there are muscle bridges between the atria and the ventricles, which can provide a conductive pathway. These muscle bridges can then provide a pathway for reentrant arrhythmias, leading to some common supraventricular arrhythmias.

Decreases in conduction through the atrioventricular bundle can lead to atrioventricular nodal block. In incomplete block, the atrioventricular node transmits only some of the atrial impulses. In complete block, there is complete dissociation between the atrial rate and the ventricular rate. The ventricular rate is then dependent on the Purkinje system, and the actual rate realized depends on the location of the ectopic pacemaker. The closer the ectopic focus is to the atrioventricular node, the higher is the rate. Ventricular rate ranges from 25 to 40 beats per minute.

The ionic basis for the cardiac action potential has best been studied in Purkinje cells and has been divided into five phases. Phase 0 is characterized by rapid membrane depolarization and reversal of the membrane potential. This is generated by the very intense, and brief, inward movement of sodium through the fast sodium channels. During this time the slow sodium-calcium channels also open. Calcium entry is important to excitation-contraction coupling. Phase 1 is the rapid repolarization to the plateau of the action potential due to inactivation of the fast sodium channels. Phase 2 is the long sustained plateau of the action potential, because the slow sodium-calcium channels have remained open. The plateau of the action potential is responsible for the fact that the duration of the action potential is about the same as that of the muscle contraction. This long duration of the action potential prevents summation and tetany in cardiac muscle. Phase 3 is the rapid repolarization to the resting potential, because of increased permeability of the membrane to potassium, and potassium exiting the cells. Phase 4 is the resting potential. The conducting cells, which possess autorhythmicity, exhibit spontaneous depolarization, so that when the potential reaches the threshold value, phase 0 depolarization is elicited. The rate of spontaneous depolarization in these cells can be altered by the autonomic nervous system—with parasympathetic stimulation decreasing the rate of depolarization and sympathetic stimulation increasing the rate of depolarization—or by disease. In ordinary atrial or ventricular muscle cells, phase 4 is a stable resting potential, which continues until the next depolarization is elicited.

ANTIARRHYTHMICS

Antiarrhythmics are classified by their cellular electrophysiologic actions (Table 5–1). The studies leading to these classifications were done in cardiac tissues isolated from experimental animals. The relationship to their clinical actions is not well understood. Dosage schedules for the antiarrhythmics are listed in Table 5–2.

Type Ia

Quinidine is derived from quinine, and its antiarrhythmic properties were discovered in treating malarial patients. Those who also had atrial fibrillation were frequently cured of that arrhythmia. Quinidine is a general cardiac depressant in that it depresses spontaneous depolarization and increases the duration of the action potential. It also depresses the conduction system, depressing ectopic foci and preventing recurrence of supraventricular tachyarrhythmias or ventricular arrhythmias. It is one of the more useful drugs for treating ventricular premature depolarization or ventricular tachycardia, and for prevention of ventricular fibrillation. Initially, it exerts an anticholinergic (decreased vagal) activity, so it may cause tachycardia. Pretreatment with digitalis prevents this from developing. Both direct and indirect actions of

TABLE 5–1.

Classification of Antiarrhythmic Drugs by Cellular Electrophysiology

Category	Mechanism	Drugs
Type I	Fast sodium channel blocking drugs	
Ia	Moderate inhibition of phase 0	Quinidine (Quinidex, others) Disopyramide (Norpace) Procainamide (Pronestyl)
Ib	Minimum inhibition of phase 0	Tocainide (Tonocard) Mexiletine (Mexitil) Lidocaine
Ic	Maximal inhibition of phase 0	Flecainide (Tambocor) Encainide (Enkaid) Propafenone (Rythmol)
Type II	Inhibition of sympathetic tone by beta adrenergic blockade (depression of phase 4 depolarization	Propranolol (Inderal) Acebutolol (Sectral)
Type III	Prolongation of repolarization (phase 3)	Amiodarone (Cordarone)
Type IV	Blockade of calcium channels; prolongation of phases 1 and 2	Verapamil (Isoptin, Calan)

TABLE 5–2.

Dosage Schedules for Antiarrhythmic Drugs

Type*	Drug	Total Daily Dose (mg)	Times/Day
Ia	Quinidine (Quinidex)	600–1,800	2–3†
	Disopyramide (Norpace)	400–600	2–4
	Procainamide (Pronestyl)	2,000–4,000	4
Ib	Tocainide (Tonocard)	1,200–1,800	3
	Mexiletine (Mexitil)	600–900	3
Ic	Flecainide (Tambocor)	300–400	2
	Encainide (Enkaid)	75–200	3
	Propafenone (Rythmol)	450–900	3
II	Propranolol (Inderal)	30–120	3–4
	Acebutolol (Sectral)	400–1,200	2
III	Amiodarone (Cordarone)	400–800	1–2
IV	Verapamil (Isoptin, Calan)	240–480	3–4

*See Table 5–1.
†Extended release.

digitalis protect against the anticholinergic effects of quinidine. Indications for use of quinidine include atrial flutter, premature atrial and ventricular contraction, paroxysmal atrioventricular junctional rhythms, paroxysmal atrial tachycardia and fibrillation, and premature ventricular tachycardia not associated with complete heart block. Quinidine also can depress skeletal and smooth muscle, causing vasodilation, leading to hypotension and skeletal muscle weakness and fatigue, especially of the respiratory muscles.

Quinidine is rapidly absorbed after oral administration, with peak serum concentrations attained in about 1 hour. It is metabolized in the liver, and the metabolites are excreted by the kidney. Its elimination half-life is 6 to 7 hours. The serum concentration of digoxin is increased in the presence of quinidine. Therefore, digoxin levels should be monitored, and the dose reduced if necessary. Also, amiodarone (Cordarone), cimetidine (Tagemet), and verapamil (Isoptin, Calan) can lead to an increased serum concentration of quinidine. Nifedipine (Procardia, Adalat), on the other hand, can lead to a decreased serum concentration of quinidine.

One third of patients using quinidine will experience adverse reactions that necessitate discontinuance. It has a low therapeutic index, so constant monitoring of the patient for adverse reactions is required. Side effects related to the gastrointestinal system, such as nausea, vomiting, and diarrhea, can be minimized if the drug is administered with food. Cinchonism is seen as tinnitus, loss of hearing, headache, and altered vision. Cardiotoxicity to quinidine is seen in the electrocardiogram, with prolonged PR intervals and a widening of the QRS complex, which is due to decreased atrioventricular conduction. There may be sinoatrial block, atrioventricular block, and ventricular tachyarrhythmias. Conduction is slowed in all parts of the heart. The Purkinje fibers can become depolarized and develop abnormal automaticity. There is a need to differentiate drug toxicity from worsening of the arrhythmia. Quinidine allows for premature beats. There may be a paradoxical increase in ventricular rate with a decrease in atrial rate. There is a risk of arterial embolism after atrial fibrillation, resulting in a stroke. Blood dyscrasias, such as thrombocytopenia, although rare, may be fatal. Hypotension is caused by relaxation of vascular smooth muscle. Anticholinergic actions may cause tachycardia. Toxicity of quinidine is increased with potassium supplementation. This is an important consideration in patients who are also prescribed a potassium-losing diuretic and potassium supplementation.

Type Ib

Lidocaine is the prototype of type Ib drugs; however, it is not effective orally, and must be given by the intravenous or intramuscular route.

Tocainide (Tonocard) is absorbed from the gastrointestinal tract, with peak blood levels attained 60 to 90 minutes after administration. It is metabolized by the liver and the metabolites are excreted by the kidneys. Its half-life is about 15 hours. Tocainide has no interaction with digoxin.

Tocainide is effective in prophylaxis and treatment of ventricular arrhythmias that develop subsequent to a myocardial infarction. It acts to suppress chronic complex ventricular ectopic beats and to prevent malignant ventricular tachyarrhythmias. It has no effect on atrial fibrillation or flutter. This drug acts to shorten the effective refractory period of the ventricle and shortens the action potential duration. It has little effect on sinus node automaticity or intracardiac conduction. It suppresses premature ventricular beats. In combination with Ia agents, such as quinidine, there is additional efficacy in 15% to 35% of patients with ventricular arrhythmias. Combination therapy with smaller doses of both drugs is often associated with lower incidence of toxicity.

Adverse effects are noted in about 40% of patients, requiring drug discontinuance in about half of these. Side effects seen with tocainide use are mainly gastrointestinal or neurologic. The gastrointestinal problems are anorexia, nausea, vomiting, abdominal pain, and constipation. Neurologic problems are tremors, nervousness, dizziness, parathesias, and mental confusion. These may be minimized if the drug is taken after meals. About 8% of patients using tocainide will develop a rash that resolves on discontinuance of the drug. There is a rare occurrence of pulmonary fibrosis or agranulocytosis (less than 0.05%). Drug-aggravated heart failure or arrhythmias are seen in less than 4% of patients. Although there is a narrow toxic to therapeutic ratio, it is generally well tolerated in patients with heart failure. This drug has no value in treatment of supraventricular arrhythmias.

Type Ic

The class Ic agents, flecainide (Tambocor) and encainide (Enkaid), prolong the refractory period and slow conduction in the atria, atrioventricular node, His-Purkinje system and ventricles, and accessory pathways. These drugs are metabolized primarily by the liver and excreted by the kidneys. Peak blood levels are attained within 2 to 4 hours after oral administration, and the half-lives are about 20 hours. Drugs in this class are effective in decreasing the frequency of premature ventricular contractions in patients with ventricular ectopy. They suppress premature ventricular contractions, ventricular couplets, and runs of nonsustained ventricular tachycardia. These agents have negative inotropic activity and depress left ventricular function and may cause or aggravate heart failure in patients. These agents are also proarrhythmic and may worsen sinus nodal function, and because of potent effects on slowing His-Purkinje conduction, may aggravate preexisting conduction disturbances and precipitate development of advanced atrioventricular block. Side effects are seen in about 30% of patients, requiring drug discontinuance in about 15%. Noncardiac side effects are dizziness, visual disturbances, dyspnea, nausea, fatigue, tremor, and headache.

Propafenone (Rythmol) is also a beta blocker and has membrane stabilizing activity. Its half-life ranges from 2 to 12 hours. It has been shown to be effective in controlling premature ventricular contractions, couplets, and nonsustained ventricular tachycardia in patients with potentially lethal ventricular arrhythmias. It prolongs the QRS interval. Because it prolongs refractoriness and slows conduction in atria, atrioventricular node, and accessory atrioventricular connections, it may be effective in patients with reentrant supraventricular tachycardia and paroxysmal atrial tachycardia.

Subjective adverse affects to propafenone are dose dependent and include a bitter, metallic taste; nausea; vomiting; and dizziness. A drug-induced rash is seen in about 3% of patients. Because of its beta-blocking activity, it can accentuate atrioventricular nodal block. Because of its Ic effects, it can aggravate His-Purkinje block. It has some negative inotropic activity and should be used with caution in patients with left ventricular dysfunction, as symptoms may worsen. Propafenone has some proarrhythmic activity, especially in patients with a history of ventricular tachycardia or ventricular fibrillation. The cardiac side effects are dose dependent and are most often seen in patients with advanced underlying disease.

Propafenone (Rythmol) does interact with digoxin and can increase digoxin levels 40% to 60%. It also appears to increase plasma concentrations of warfarin, and thus increases prothrombin times.

Flecainide (Tambocor) and encainide (Enkaid) have shown excess mortality among patients with nonsustained ventricular arrhythmias after a myocardial infarction. The U.S. Food and Drug Administration has relabeled both as indicated only in patients with documented ventricular arrhythmias such as sustained ventricular tachycardia that are life-threatening. Propafenone (Rythmol) has the same labeling.

Type II

Beta blockers block the interaction of epinephrine and norepinephrine with beta receptors and inhibit the actions of these catecholamines on the heart. Beta blockers are useful in supraventricular arrhythmias, atrial fibrillation, atrial flutter, and paroxysmal atrial tachycardia. Because of increased refractoriness of the atrioventricular node, they slow conduction in the atrioventricular node. Thus, they slow ventricular rate rather than abolish the arrhythmia. Propranolol (Inderal) is beneficial for treatment of arrhythmias induced by exercise or emotions, when the sympathetic nervous system is implicated. Propranolol has been shown to reduce death and nonfatal myocardial infarction in the first year after a first myocardial infarction, and it increases the threshold for ventricular fibrillation after a myocardial infarction. Propranolol and digitalis are additive in treatment of atrial fibrillation and atrial flutter. Digitalis increases vagal tone, and propranolol is a beta blocker.

Long-term blockade causes an adaptational response in heart cells that delays repolarization. This effect takes weeks to develop, reaches a plateau in about 3 weeks, and persists for days after cessation of treatment.

Acebutolol (Sectral) is a relatively cardioselective beta-1 blocker, which has been approved for management of ventricular arrhythmias. It is more cardioselective than propranolol and also has partial agonist activity. It causes less reduction in heart rate than propranolol, but slows atrioventricular conduction and prolongs atrioventricular nodal refractoriness. The half-life of acebutolol and its major metabolites is 8 to 13 hours. It can be effective in paroxysmal supraventricular tachycardia and atrial fibrillation, partially by slowing atrioventricular nodal conduction. Beta blockers have low proarrhythmic activity, and may be the drug of choice in exercise-induced ventricular tachycardia. They are useful for digitalis-induced arrhythmias and symptoms associated with the mitral valve prolapse syndrome.

Adverse effects, similar to other beta blockers, are depression and fatigue. Asthma and other bronchospastic diseases can be exacerbated. Worsening of atrioventricular nodal block and aggravation of heart failure due to negative inotropy also may occur.

Type III

Amiodarone (Cordarone) has many properties, but is classified as type III because it prolongs repolarization. Its principal effect is to prolong the QT interval but it also prolongs the PR interval and prolongs the action potential duration. It also has coronary and peripheral vasodilating properties. Amiodarone is slowly and variably absorbed after oral administration. Its half-life is about 53 days, so it takes months to reach equilibrium. It is metabolized in the liver, so renal impairment does not necessitate a dose reduction. This agent has been approved for treatment of life-threatening ventricular arrhythmias. It is useful in treatment of sustained ventricular tachycardia, which is refractory to other drugs. Amiodarone is indicated for recurrent ventricular fibrillation and recurrent ventricular tachycardia. Because of its long half-life and end-organ toxicity, it is not a first-line drug. Indications for its use are recurrent ventricular fibrillation and recurrent ventricular tachycardia.

Although adverse effects to amiodarone are common, they require drug withdrawal in less than 20% of patients. Listed as minor effects are corneal microdeposits, asymptomatic transient elevation of hepatic enzymes, photosensitivity of skin (use sun screens and other protection from the sun), bluish-gray skin discolorations, and subjective gastrointestinal side effects such as nausea, vomiting, anorexia, and constipation, which may respond to dose reduction. This agent may induce hypothyroidism, which requires thyroid replacement. It paradoxically may induce hyperthyroidism, which requires discontinuance of the drug. More serious effects are interstitial pneumonitis, which is usually reversible on discontinuance of the drug, and drug-induced hepatitis. Neurologic effects include peripheral neuropathy and myopathy, malaise and fatigue, tremor and involuntary movements, and ataxia; all usually resolve on dose reduction.

Amiodarone has minimal negative inotropy. However, it does interact with digoxin, warfarin (Coumadin), quinidine, procainamide (Pronestyl), mexiletine (Mexitil), and flecainide (Tambocor). Digoxin levels double, prothrombin time doubles or triples, and blood levels of class I agents increase 15% to 35%. Concomitant use requires lower doses and close monitoring.

Type IV

Calcium channel blockers inhibit entry of calcium into arterial smooth muscle, myocytes, and cardiac conduction cells. They are used in treatment of supraventricular arrhythmias, such as atrial flutter or fibrillation. They act by slowing the firing rate of the sinoatrial node and by decreasing conduction velocity through the atrioventricular node. Thus, they decrease ventricular rate at rest.

Of the calcium channel blockers, only verapamil (Isoptin, Calan) is approved for antiarrhythmic therapy. It has a rapid onset of action and is metabolized by the liver. Dosage reduction may be necessary in chronic liver disease, if the half-life is increased. In the presence of renal disease, on the other hand, no change in dosing is required. It is generally well tolerated. In the elderly who may show increased susceptibility to sinoatrial depression, fatigue, constipation, and hypotension, lower doses and less frequent intervals of dosing may be necessary. However, because of its mechanism of action, verapamil should not be used with preexisting left ventricular dysfunction. It may lead to a decrease in contractility and a further decrease in left ventricular function. With normal left ventricular function, however, there seems to be no compromise in left ventricular function. A small percentage of users will have headaches from cerebral vascular dilation, dizziness, and gastrointestinal symptoms, such as constipation, due to decreased gastrointestinal smooth muscle activity. Preexisting atrioventricular nodal conduction disturbances may be exacerbated.

Verapamil (Isoptin, Calan) is indicated for use in prophylaxis of repetitive paroxysmal atrial tachycardia. It prolongs the effective refractory period within the atrioventricular node and slows conduction. It thus slows ventricular rate in atrial flutter or fibrillation.

Verapamil is also indicated for treatment of essential hypertension and of angina pectoris, at rest. Its use in these indications is further discussed in Chapters 4 and 6.

PHYSICAL THERAPY NOTES

The advantage of continuous monitoring for arrhythmias during cardiac rehabilitation is obvious. Monitoring of arrhythmias without continuous monitoring is not easy. Many arrhythmias are not readily discerned by palpation alone.

Sympathetic nervous system stimulation, such as from mental stress or exercise, can induce arrhythmias in susceptible individuals.

LEARNING OBJECTIVES

1. Understand the physiology of the cardiac rhythm.
2. Describe the pharmacology of the various classes of antiarrhythmic drugs and relate that to the types of arrhythmias that are amenable to treatment by the different classes of drugs.
3. Explain the cardiac and noncardiac side effects of the various classes of antiarrhythmics.

ADDITIONAL READINGS

1. Benditt DG, Goldstein MA, Reyes WJ, et al: Supraventricular tachycardias: Mechanisms and therapies. *Hosp Pract* 1988; 23(Aug):161–185.
2. Funck-Brentano C, Kroemer HK, Lee JT, et al: Propafenone. *N Engl J Med* 1990; 322:518–525.
3. Kreeger RW, Hammill SC: New antiarrhythmic drugs: Tocainide, mexiletine, flecainide, encainide, and amiodarone. *Mayo Clin Proc* 1987; 62:1033–1050.

4. Naccarelli GV, Rinkenberger RL, Dougherty AH, et al: Pharmacologic therapy of arrhythmias. *Hosp Pract* 1988; 23(Oct):183–210.
5. Petersen P: Thromboembolic complications of atrial fibrillation and their prevention: A review. *Am J Cardiol* 1990; 65:24C–28C.
6. Ravid S, Podrid PJ, Lampert S, et al: Congestive heart failure induced by six of the newer antiarrhythmic drugs. *J Am Coll Cardiol* 1989; 14:1326–1330.
7. Vaughan Williams EM: Relevance of cellular to clinical electrophysiology in interpreting antiarrhythmic drug action. *Am J Cardiol* 1989; 64:5J–9J.
8. Vaughan Williams EM: Classification of antiarrhythmic actions, in Vaughan Williams EM (ed): *Handbook of Experimental Pharmacology,* vol 89. Berlin, Springer-Verlag, 1989, pp 45–67.

Chapter 6

Drugs Used in Treatment of Vascular Disease and Tissue Ischemia

Narrowing of a blood vessel lumen causes a decrease in blood flow delivery to tissues. This eventually leads to ischemia, or inadequate blood flow necessary to maintain normal function of the tissues. Physiologic responses to decreased blood flow and, therefore, to reduced oxygen delivery, are vasodilation, due to autoregulation, and angiogenesis or formation of new blood vessels. Vasodilation may maintain suitable blood flow delivery if the amount of narrowing is not too great. Angiogenesis occurs over a protracted time period and may allow appropriate blood delivery through new channels if the development of occlusion is slow. The narrowed vessel, besides causing ischemia itself, can cause activation of hemostatic mechanisms, platelet activation, and blood clotting, which can then further occlude vessels and reduce flow.

VASCULAR DISEASE

Atherosclerosis

Arteriosclerosis is a general term for pathologic thickening and hardening of the arterial wall. Atherosclerosis more specifically refers to this process in the larger arteries. These vascular changes are responsible for coronary artery disease, cerebral artery disease, and peripheral artery disease. There are changes in vessel walls with aging, but these are separate and distinct from those seen with arteriosclerosis. With aging, there is a slow and continuous symmetric increase in the thickness of the intima, the inner layer of the vessel wall. Smooth muscle cells accumulate and are surrounded by connective tissue. The lipid content of the vessel wall, especially cholesterol esters and phospholipids, increases with age. The cholesterol esters that accumulate in the intima are derived from the plasma.

Atherosclerosis is considered by many to be an inflammatory process, with three phenomena: lipid accumulation, smooth muscle proliferation, and eventually vessel occlusion. Injury to the intimal layer causes loss of endothelial cells and exposes the subendothelial connective tissue to circulating platelets. The activation and aggregation of platelets cause release of platelets factors that further induce smooth muscle and endothelial proliferation. Lipid infiltration and fibroblast proliferation lead to the sclerosis and occlusion of the vessel. Downstream from the occlusion, the velocity of blood flow decreases, which may allow for thrombus (clot) formation. Part of the thrombus may break free and form an embolus, a free-floating thrombus. The embolus can travel in the blood until it reaches a vessel smaller than it can pass through, which it then occludes. Risk factors for atherogenesis that are capable of producing chronic injury to the arterial wall are the increased shear stress of hypertension and the metabolic derangements from hypercholesterolemia, hypertriglyceridemia, and hyperglycemia. Vascular problems are more common in diabetics. In addition to involvement of large arteries, there is a disease of the small arteries seen specifically in diabetics. This small vessel disease involves thickening of the vessel wall, especially in the feet.

Cholesterol Metabolism

Cholesterol and triglycerides are transported in plasma in lipoproteins. The lipoproteins differ from one another in size and density and in relative proportions of triglycerides and cholesterol esters. The liver secretes triglycerides into the plasma in very low-density lipoproteins (VLDLs), which are then degraded to low-density lipoproteins (LDLs) by lipoprotein lipase, an enzyme that is bound to the inner surface of blood vessels. The lipoprotein lipase removes the triglycerides from the VLDLs, and the triglycerides are then taken up by cells. The remaining LDLs can be taken up by the liver or extrahepatic cells when cholesterol is needed for membrane synthesis. This uptake of LDLs requires the presence of LDL receptors on the cells. Synthesis of LDL receptors is regulated by the cholesterol need of the cell. Cells also can synthesize their own cholesterol; 3-hydroxy-3-methylglutaryl coenzyme A (HMG-CoA) reductase is the rate-limiting enzyme in the synthesis of cholesterol. The involvement of LDL-cholesterol in atherogenesis has been well documented in clinical and pathologic studies, as well as in many animal experiments. High LDL levels are a risk factor for development of atherosclerosis. Another type of lipoprotein, the high-density lipoproteins (HDLs), are involved in the removal of cholesterol from tissues ("reverse transport"). Also, of clinical importance is the HDL level, and its ratio to LDL. Other risk factors that can be modified are weight, diet, smoking, exercise level, and control of diabetes mellitus.

Initial treatment of hypercholesterolemia includes cessation of smoking, weight loss if necessary, diet modification to one low in cholesterol, low in total fat, low in saturated fat, and relatively high in unsaturated fat; an increased exercise level; and control of diabetes mellitus, if applicable. In patients with mild elevation of blood cholesterol, these nonpharmacologic modifications should be attempted for 3 to 6 months. Because treatment of the hyperlipidemias is a lifelong effort, patient compliance is important.

HEMOSTASIS

Platelets

Platelets, or thrombocytes, are incomplete cells, formed from pinching off membrane and cytoplasm of megakaryocytes. They normally circulate in the blood in a quiescent state and, unless stimulated, have a life span of about 10 days. Maintenance of the unreactive state is due to both lack of reactive stimuli and the inhibitory action of prostacyclin released from intact endothelial cells lining the blood vessels. Platelet reactivity is promoted by an absence of prostacyclin secretion from damaged endothelial cells and by certain stimuli, such as rough surfaces on the inner wall of the blood vessel and certain chemicals such as thromboxane and serotonin released from activated platelets.

Stimulated platelets undergo processes of activation and aggregation. Platelets release chemicals that contract smooth muscle and activate other platelets. They also become sticky on the outer surface of the membrane and stick to each other and to damaged endothelium. These processes are important in formation of the platelet plug at the site of endothelial injury. The platelet plug serves to protect the injured endothelium while repair processes take place.

Platelet plug formation is a positive-feedback cycle and occurs as a local reaction at the site of injury. Localization of the platelet plug to the site of injury is important; otherwise, each endothelial injury would activate all the platelets in the body. Localization is maintained by the velocity of the blood in the vessel, moving most of the blood past the injury site more rapidly than the platelets can be activated. Also, an intact endothelium in noninjured areas inhibits platelet activation.

Blood Clot Formation

Clotting factors are proteins that are synthesized in the liver and circulate in an inactive form. Stimulation of the process of blood clotting occurs when there is a break in the vessel wall and exposure of the clotting factors to collagen within the vessel wall. The first clotting factor, factor XII (Hageman factor) is activated, which initiates the clotting process, sequentially activating the proteins in the cascade. Figure 6–1 shows a schemata of the clotting cascade. Each active factor acts as a proteolytic enzyme, and cleaves the inactive fragment from the next factor, again forming an active enzyme. This sequence occurs until the last active factor, fibrin, is formed. Fibrin is a structural protein that forms a meshlike network, trapping cells and platelets. Platelets are activated during this time and, as part of their reactivity, form pseudopods that intermingle with the fibrin. Retraction of the pseudopods, "clot retraction," causes the formation of a firmer, more stable clot.

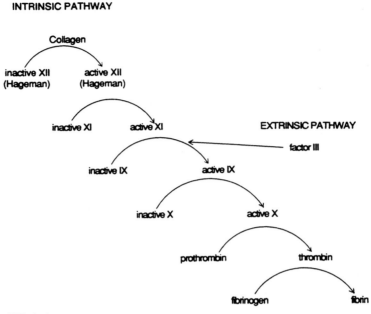

INTRINSIC PATHWAY

FIG 6–1.
Schematic drawing of the blood clotting cascade. The *intrinsic pathway* is initiated in the blood; the *extrinsic pathway* is initiated in the extravascular space. Activation of each factor in sequence forms a proteolytic enzyme, which activates the next factor. The cascade must occur in sequence. Lack of any factor, such as in hemophilia, prevents culmination of the cascade and thus prevents blood clotting.

At the same time the clotting cascade is occurring, a slower process, which will finally result in clot dissolution, is initiated. Whereas clot formation is rapid, within minutes, clot dissolution will occur over a period of a week. Active factor XII (Hageman factor) also causes the transformation of plasminogen to plasmin, which will proteolytically break down the fibrin network. After the clot has formed, processes to repair the injury to the vessel wall begin. These repair processes should be well under way by the time the clot dissolutes.

Clot formation is another positive feedback cycle occurring at the site of injury. Tissue factors released due to an injury are also involved. Localization to the site of injury is again maintained by the velocity of blood in the vessel and the presence of an intact endothelium inhibiting clot formation. Inappropriate clotting can occur if the velocity of blood flow is sufficiently slow to allow for interaction of the fibrin. This occurs in situations of venous stasis, such as in varicose veins or in atrial fibrillation.

Pharmacologic treatment of atherosclerotic disease once it has developed has not proved very successful, owing to the long-term development of the disease. So far, we do not have drugs that will reverse atherosclerosis already present. However, some recent reports have demonstrated possible reversal with dietary and pharmacologic management. Prevention is, by far, the better course. Reduction of reversible risk factors is encouraged, with smoking cessation, weight reduction, control of hypertension, and control of hyperlipidemias and hyperglycemia recommended. Other general treatments of vascular disease involve attempts to make the blood less likely to form both fibrin clots and platelet plugs, using the so-called "blood thinners."

In this chapter the treatments for generalized atherosclerosis, the lipid-lowering agents, the antithrombotics, and the anticoagulants are discussed first. Later, drugs more specific for the localized symptoms, coronary artery disease, cerebrovascular disease, and peripheral vascular disease are presented.

LIPID-LOWERING AGENTS

Bile Acid Binding Resins

The oldest class of lipid-lowering agents is the bile acid binding resins, which bind bile acids in the lumen of the intestinal tract. Cholestyramine (Questran, Cholybar) and colestipol (Colestid) are the two resins available in the United States. The resin forms a nonabsorbable complex with the bile acids that inhibits their reabsorption from the intestinal lumen. The bound bile acids are then excreted with the resin in the feces. Bile acids are synthesized in the liver from cholesterol. So this inhibition of bile acid reabsorption increases liver production of bile acids from cholesterol. This in turn lowers plasma LDL-cholesterol and thus increases hepatic and extrahepatic receptors for LDL, which increases uptake of LDL from the plasma. When used as monotherapy, these agents cause a 5% to 20% lowering of blood cholesterol levels. Triglycerides may increase or stay the same. The resins have an excellent efficacy and safety record. Because they are not absorbed from the gastrointestinal tract, systemic side effects are avoided. There may be abdominal discomfort, which can, however, limit compliance. There is also impairment of absorption of fat-soluble vitamins. Bleeding disorders may result from decreased absorption of vitamin K, which is required for synthesis of clotting factors. The resin also may bind other drugs in the intestinal tract, thus limiting their absorption. This interaction is especially important in decreasing absorption of warfarin, chlorothiazide, phenylbutazone, propranolol, digitalis, and phenobarbital. These interactions can be avoided if the other drugs are taken at least 1 hour before or 4 to 6 hours after the resin. Cholestyramine is available as the resin (Questran), which must be mixed with liquid, and as a bar (Cholybar). Dosages of these are listed in Table 6–1. The sandy or gritty quality of the resin may limit compliance.

Nicotinic Acid

Nicotinic acid (niacin), by an unknown mechanism of action, decreases liver production of VLDL, thereby reducing the plasma levels of VLDL-cholesterol and triglycerides by 20% to 80%, and LDL-cholesterol by 10% to 15%. This drug is

TABLE 6–1.

Lipid Lowering Agents

Drug	Total Daily Dose	Times/Day
Resins		
Cholestyramine (Questran, Cholybar)	4–24 g	1–6
Colestipol (Colestid)	15–30 g	2–4
Nicotinic acid		
Nicolar	3–6 g	3
Nia-Bid (sustained release)	1,200–2,400 mg	3
Nicobid (timed release)	250–1,000 mg	2
Fibric acid derivatives		
Gemfibrozil (Lopid)	1,200 mg	2
Clofibrate (Atromid-S)	2 g	2–4
Probucol (Lorelco)	1,000 mg	2
HMG-CoA reductase inhibitors		
Lovastatin (Mevacor)	20–80 mg	1

more commonly used in conjunction with a bile acid binding resin, the combination of which causes further reductions in VLDL cholesterol and triglyceride levels. The most common adverse reaction to nicotinic acid is cutaneous flushing and itching. The flushing may be blocked with aspirin. It is aggravated by alcohol and hot beverages. Nicotinic acid administered with an alpha blocker may produce postural hypotension. Glucose tolerance may be reduced in diabetic patients. Because of its side effects, nicotinic acid is not so well tolerated as some other lipid lowering drugs. Taking the drug with meals may alleviate some problems. Nicotinic acid preparations are listed in Table 6–1.

Fibric acid derivatives

Clofibrate (Atromid-S) decreases plasma levels of VLDL and triglycerides through mechanisms that decrease production of, and increase removal of, VLDL. These actions then lead to a decreased VLDL-triglyceride and VLDL levels, as well as a more variable action on cholesterol and LDL. Lipoprotein lipase activity is increased, which accounts, in part, for the decrease in VLDL levels. This agent is less effective than others that lower cholesterol. Adverse reactions are most commonly nausea, diarrhea, and a flulike syndrome with cramps and weakness. It may cause development of gall stones and liver tumors. When used in combination with anticoagulants, there is increased risk of bleeding. The anticoagulant dose should then be reduced.

Gemfibrozil (Lopid) causes reduced triglyceride and VLDL levels, with a variable effect on LDL. It also raises HDL, so the ratio of LDL to HDL is improved. The fibric acid derivatives are listed in Table 6–1.

Probucol

Probucol (Lorelco) lowers LDL cholesterol 10% to 20%, but the response is variable. This drug acts through a non-LDL receptor mechanism, so is effective in those patients without LDL receptors. It, however, lowers HDL, so has an unfavorable action on the LDL to HDL ratio. Dosage for probucol is listed in Table 6–1.

Cholesterol Synthesis Inhibition

Lovastatin (Mevacor) is a specific inhibitor of HMG-CoA reductase, the rate-limiting step in cholesterol synthesis in the liver. It has a spectrum of action similar to that of the resins, with a decrease in LDL, and a small increase in HDL. Its inhibitory action on intracellular cholesterol synthesis is responsible for the increased LDL receptor activity. Lovastatin is a pro-drug, and is activated in the liver to the active form. It is carried in the blood tightly bound to plasma proteins. Although its half-life is 1 to 2 hours, clinical trials have indicated a once or twice daily dosing regimen is sufficient for therapeutic efficacy. A single dose given in the evening even may be sufficient, because cholesterol is mainly synthesized at night. Although a clinical effect is evident in 2 weeks, a maximum effect takes 4 to 6 weeks to develop. Dosage for lovastatin is listed in Table 6–1. It is metabolized in the liver and excreted in the bile, and should therefore be used with caution in patients with impaired liver function or taking hepatotoxic drugs. It is used as an adjunct to diet for reduction of elevated total and LDL cholesterol levels in patients with primary hypercholesterolemia when their response to diet, exercise, and weight reduction has been inadequate. Its effects are additive with the bile acid binding resin cholestyramine, causing a cholesterol lowering of greater than 50%. It is well tolerated acutely. Its side effects seem to be minor and of no greater incidence than with placebos. Rarely, a reversible myopathy may be seen. It was licensed in the United States in 1987, so its long-term use is still under investigation. Two similarly acting drugs, simvastatin and pravastatin, although not yet approved by the FDA, are in clinical studies in North America and Europe.

Combination therapy using a bile acid binding resin plus a systemic agent, such as niacin, gemfibrozil, or lovastatin, shows an additive or synergistic reduction in total and LDL-cholesterol, without a drug interaction. Combination therapy may cause an efficacy similar to that of higher doses of either drug alone; it allows for lower doses in combination, with a reduction in side effects. This is especially true of the resins, where the total dose required in monotherapy causes sufficient problems to the patient, and thus reduces compliance.

ANTITHROMBOTICS, ANTICOAGULANTS, AND THROMBOLYTICS

Anticoagulants and antithrombotics are frequently used in treatment of occlusive vascular diseases. Normally, blood clotting and platelet aggregation are inhibited because of the smooth endothelial lining of the cardiovascular system. Loss or disruption of the smooth surface can cause activation of clotting factors and platelet aggregation.

Antithrombotics

The nonsteroidal anti-inflammatory agents, aspirin and others, irreversibly inhibit platelet aggregation, but do not change the number of circulating platelets. The antithrombotic duration of action of aspirin is 10 days, until new platelets are formed. This treatment is used in recurrent myocardial infarction and in strokes (transient ischemic attacks), to prevent or minimize the next occurrence. Current recommendations are one-half to one regular aspirin a day. This low level rarely causes gastrointestinal problems. Dipyridamole (Persantine) is used in post-valve replacement patients (with warfarin). Sulfinpyrazone (Anturane) inhibits platelet function; however, the FDA has not approved it for this use. The nonsteroidal anti-inflammatory agents are further discussed in Chapter 14.

Anticoagulants

Anticoagulants inhibit the clotting factors, thus they prevent clot formation but do not lyse clots already formed. They prevent not only formation of new clots, but also extension of clots already formed. Heparin is a naturally occurring anticoagulant, but its physiologic significance is not understood. It cannot be given orally, which limits its outpatient use. Heparin inhibits preformed clotting factors, so its onset of action is immediate. Since heparin is an animal extract, allergic reactions may occur. Overdose of heparin is managed by immediately withdrawing the heparin. Heparin has a short half-life, so it is rapidly removed from the body.

The oral anticoagulant warfarin (Coumadin) was first used as a rodenticide. This drug acts in the liver to inhibit synthesis of the clotting factors. It has a slower onset of action than heparin, of over a day, and a longer duration of action. Because warfarin is a vitamin K antagonist, treatment of overdosage involves administration of massive amounts of vitamin K to overcome the inhibition.

Bleeding, the major adverse effect of anticoagulant use, is dose related. Nosebleeds, gum bleeding, and small areas of bleeding into the skin may be seen. Because massive hemorrhage may occur with injury, extreme care must be used when handling patients, as even minor trauma may result in severe hemorrhage. The risk of bleeding is increased with concurrent use of antiplatelet drugs, such as aspirin.

Many drug interactions with warfarin may be due to increased activity because of plasma protein displacement by other drugs. The dose of warfarin may need to be reduced, as the free drug concentration is important. Displacement from plasma proteins will cause a decrease in duration of action, so it may need to be administered more frequently, at lower doses. The toxicity of warfarin is also increased when used in combination with drugs that inhibit platelet activity, such as aspirin and other nonsteroidal anti-inflammatory agents. Acetaminophen can be used as a replacement for aspirin in treatment of fever and pain. Warfarin activity may be increased in liver disease, because of decreased metabolism of the oral anticoagulants. Also, warfarin activity may be decreased due to increased liver metabolism with concomitant use of barbiturates.

Thrombolytics

Thrombolytics promote dissolution of thrombi by activating plasmin formation. The drugs currently available for this purpose are streptokinase and tissue plasminogen activator (TPA). These are used immediately after a myocardial infarction in an attempt to dissolve the clot and promote blood flow into the ischemic area.

ISCHEMIC HEART DISEASE

Angina pectoris is pain associated with decreased blood flow necessary for cardiac muscle contraction. In other words, angina is a situation of either an increase in oxygen demand or a decrease in oxygen supply. Angina is the principal symptom of ischematic heart disease, starting substernally, and radiating to the left shoulder and flexor surface of the left arm. It can be induced by exercise, emotions, or eating. Silent myocardial ischemia, by definition, does not result in clinical symptoms. The reason for the lack of symptoms with verified ischemia is unknown. Angina is associated with ST depression on the electrocardiogram. Frequently, the decreased blood flow is due to atherosclerosis of the coronary arteries. However, in those patients with normal coronary arteries, variant angina (Prinzmetal's) is due to vasospasm at rest associated with ST elevation. Increased blood flow can be affected by dilation of the coronary arteries to increase flow to the heart, dilation of peripheral arterioles to decrease work of the heart (decreased afterload), or dilation of veins to decrease venous return (decreased preload), and thus decrease stroke volume, and decrease work of the heart.

There are three classes of drugs currently used to treat angina pectoris: nitrates, beta blockers, and calcium channel blockers.

Nitrates

Nitroglycerin has been used since the 1880s. It dilates arterioles (reduces afterload) and veins (reduces preload); however, it has a greater effect on veins. Nitroglycerin decreases end diastolic pressure more than it decreases systemic arterial pressure. Heart rate is generally unchanged, so there is a decreased cardiac output. Also, this agent has a dilatory effect on the large coronary arteries. With sublingual administration, the onset of action is within 1 to 3 minutes, and may persist up to 30 minutes. It is used for acute attacks and prophylactically in anticipation of exercise or stress. Nitroglycerin is rapidly and totally inactivated in the liver, so sublingual administration bypasses that organ of metabolism (i.e., avoid first-pass metabolism).

A longer acting oral preparation, isosorbide dinitrate (Isordil), is available, which should provide longer protection. There is also a skin patch, containing nitroglycerin (Transderm-Nitro), which slowly releases the drug, which is then absorbed through the skin. There is a possibility that a person will develop tolerance to the effects of

TABLE 6–2.

Beta Blockers

Drug	Total Daily Dose (mg)	Times/Day
Mixed beta blockers		
Propranolol (Inderal)	80–320*	2–4
	180–240†	2–3
Nadolol (Corgard)	40–80*	1
Timolol (Blocadren)	20†	2
Beta-1 blockers		
Atenolol (Tenormin)	50–200*	1
Metoprolol (Lopressor)	100–400*	2
	200†	2

*Angina.
†Myocardial infarction.

the nitrates with continuous exposure. In order to provide a drug-free time and protect the person against angina, intermittent therapy is advocated. This means using the skin patch for 12 to 14 hours, or taking isosorbide during the day, with the last dose at dinner rather than before bedtime. Tolerance does not develop with intermittent therapy of the sublingually administered nitroglycerin.

Adverse reactions to nitroglycerin are headache, because of dilation of cerebral vessels, and dizziness, weakness, and possibly fainting, all due to hypotension. The person should sit down and reduce physical activity before administering nitroglycerin to prevent cerebral ischemia.

Beta Blockers

Beta blockers are effective against exertional angina. They are not used for spastic angina; in fact they may worsen that situation. Beta blockers reduce systolic pressure and heart rate, both components of the "double product" (systolic pressure × heart rate), an indication of myocardial oxygen demand. Beta blockers with intrinsic sympathomimetic activity cause little slowing of heart rate and little depression of contractility at rest, but block exercise-induced increases in both heart rate and contractility. This may be of advantage to those persons with sympathetically mediated angina. Propranolol (Inderal) should be used with extreme caution or not at all in patients with respiratory conditions, with compromised left ventricular function, or with diabetes mellitus. The beta blockers are listed in Table 6–2 with specific doses for angina and after a myocardial infarction.

The combination of a beta blocker and a nitrate prevents the reflex tachycardia caused by the nitrate. Beta blockers are also effective antihypertensive agents. Beta blockers have been shown to prevent reinfarction and prolong life after an acute myocardial infarction. For a more complete discussion of beta blockers, see Chapter 4, Antihypertensive Drugs.

TABLE 6–3

Calcium Channel Blockers

Drug	Total Daily Dose (mg)	Times/Day
Verapamil (Isoptin, Calan)	120–360*	3
Diltiazem (Cardizem)	180–360*	3–4
Nifedipine (Procardia, Adalat)	30–60*	3
Nicardipine (Cardene)	60–120*	3
Nimodipine (Nimotop)	360†	6, for 21 days

*Angina.
†Stroke.

Calcium Channel Blockers

Calcium channel blockers, which act to decrease entry of calcium into cardiac and smooth muscle cells, are effective in variant (Prinzmetal's) angina. This type of angina is thought to result from coronary vessel spasm rather than atherosclerotic occlusive disease. Calcium channel blockers are useful in treating effort-induced angina, when beta blockers are ineffective or contraindicated. When beta blockers are contraindicated, such as in left ventricular dysfunction or sick sinus syndrome, a calcium channel blocker may be used. In these patients, nifedipine is used rather than one of the others, because it has less of a depressant action of contractility and conduction. Calcium channel blockers are also effective for both hypertension and angina. The calcium channel blockers are listed in Table 6–3. For a more complete discussion of the calcium channel blockers, see Chapter 4, Antihypertensive Drugs.

CEREBRAL ISCHEMIA

Stroke can result from hemorrhage from a cerebral vessel or blockage of a cerebral vessel, with subsequent ischemia and infarction. Cerebral vessel blockage is the most common cause of stroke. Blockage of a vessel can be from an atheromatous plaque, a thrombus forming over a plaque, or an embolus. Transient ischemic attacks (TIAs) refer to sudden neurologic deficits that clear within several hours. They are thought to be due to intermittent reductions in blood flow and usually forewarn of a stroke. Generally, atheromatous plaques form at vessel branchings. If sufficient vessel lumen narrowing occurs, blood flow velocity distal to the narrowing may be decreased and allow for thrombus formation. Cerebral embolism is the most common cause of ischemic stroke, and the heart is the most common source of emboli. Thrombus formation due to atrial fibrillation, valvular heart disease, prosthetic valves, or myocardial infarction can lead to distant embolization. Neurologic signs and symptoms and the temporal profile of these can suggest the location of the ischemic area. In ischemic stroke, collateral circulation may reduce the size of, or prevent, infarction.

Pharmacologic treatment of cerebrovascular disease has utilized some of the knowledge, and drugs, used to treat coronary artery disease. However, randomized, controlled studies are needed to show the efficacy of these treatments.

During an evolving stroke, a "stroke in progress," when symptoms are fluctuating, acute use of heparin for anticoagulation may be warranted. Chronic anticoagulation may be maintained with warfarin.

Nimodipine (Nimotop) is a calcium blocker with a greater effect on cerebral arteries. It reduces the severity of neurologic deficits resulting from vasospasm. Its use is indicated in subarachnoid hemorrhage. See Table 6–3 for details on nimodipine use.

Aspirin has been shown to be effective in treatment of TIAs. The search for agents without the attendant side effects of aspirin continues. Ticlopidine (Ticlid) inhibits platelet function, but through a different mechanism than aspirin. Aspirin inhibits cyclooxygenase, an enzyme in the prostaglandin synthesis pathway. Ticlopidine, on the other hand, has an action on the cell membrane to block aggregation induced by adenosine diphosphate. Ticlopidine is well absorbed from the gastrointestinal tract after oral administration. It is metabolized by the liver to water-soluble products, which are excreted by the kidney. It should be used with caution, or not at all, in patients with impaired liver or kidney function.

The most commonly reported adverse effects from ticlopidine use are related to the gastrointestinal system, including diarrhea, dyspepsia, nausea, and gastrointestinal pain. Rash and neutropenia have also been reported. Severe neutropenia may occur, and is usually noted within the first 3 months of treatment. For this reason, monitoring of blood counts is recommended. The neutropenia is reversible upon discontinuation of the drug.

PERIPHERAL VASCULAR DISEASE

Atherosclerosis of the peripheral arteries, especially in the lower extremities, can cause sufficient occlusion of the vessel to impede blood flow to the muscles. This causes intermittent claudication, or pain associated with exercise. The most common location is in the femoral arteries, with the iliac and popliteal arteries following in frequency. Treatment of this type of vascular disease is not very satisfactory. Pain during exercise is associated with about 50% occlusion of the vessel. About 70% to 90% narrowing occurs before there is pain at rest, with insufficient blood flow to maintain even basal skeletal muscle oxidative metabolism. Vasodilators are generally ineffective because of the sclerosis or hardening of the vessel wall. Ischemia is itself an inducer of vasodilation, so the vessels in the ischemic area would already be maximally dilated. Dilation of vessels in the nonischemic areas may "steal" blood flow from ischemic areas. However, if the occlusion of the vessel occurs over a protracted period of time, collateral vessels may develop around the occlusion because of the angiogenic effect of ischemia. Thus, blood flow to the distal parts of the extremities may be restored. Exercise therapy has proved effective in many cases to increase the time of exercise before pain occurs.

Pentoxifylline (Trental) has been used in treatment of intermittent claudication associated with peripheral vascular disease. It improves flow properties of blood by reducing blood viscosity. Because many patients with chronic occlusive arterial disease of the limbs also have evidence of cerebral arterial disease and coronary disease, this agent may improve blood flow and oxygen delivery to these tissues as well.

PHYSICAL THERAPY NOTES

Nitroglycerin, because of its greater effect on veins than on arteries, is quite likely to cause postural hypotension. Prevention of falling after a dose of this drug is important. The patient should be instructed to sit down before administration of the drug.

Pain associated with exercise in peripheral vascular disease is usually in the calf, foot, or buttocks. The onset of pain is predictable with a fixed amount of exercise and is relieved by rest. Exercise therapy improves symptoms by unknown mechanisms. Because peripheral vascular disease frequently coexists with coronary artery disease, exercise training can be planned with both diseases in mind.

The chronic use of anticoagulants and antithrombotics poses a particular danger to their users. The anticoagulants inhibit the clotting factors, so prolonged bleeding from even a minor injury may occur. The antithrombotics inhibit platelet aggregation, and easy bruisability can occur, even from the most minor of bumps.

LEARNING OBJECTIVES

1. Understand normal vascular anatomy and physiology, and the pathophysiology of atherogenesis.
2. Know the drugs, and their mechanisms and sites of action, used in treatment of coronary artery disease.
3. Know the basic mechanisms involved in hemostasis.
4. Understand the difference in mechanisms of action between heparin and the oral anticoagulants and how this influences the pharmacology of the drugs.
5. Know the drugs that interact with the oral anticoagulants.
6. Explain the reason for use of antithrombotics in treatment of occlusive vascular disease.
7. Understand the basic physiology of cholesterol metabolism.
8. Describe the therapeutic treatments available for hypercholesterolemia, their sites of actions, and side effects.

ADDITIONAL READINGS

1. Beller GA: Calcium antagonists in the treatment of Prinzmetal's angina and unstable angina pectoris. *Circulation* 1989; 80(suppl IV):IV-78–IV-87.

2. Bowton DL, Stump DA, Prough DS, et al: Pentoxifylline increases cerebral blood flow in patients with cerebrovascular disease. *Stroke* 1989; 20:1662–1666.
3. Crawford MH: Theoretical considerations in the use of calcium entry blockers in silent myocardial ischemia. *Circulation* 1989; 80(suppl IV):IV-74–IV-77.
4. Hiatt WR, Regensteiner JG, Hargarten ME, et al: Benefit of exercise conditioning for patients with peripheral arterial disease. *Circulation* 1990; 81:602–609.
5. LaRose JC, Hunninghake D, Bush D, et al: The cholesterol facts. A joint statement by the American Heart Association and the National Heart, Lung, and Blood Institute. *Circulation* 1990; 81:1721–1733.
6. McTavish D, Faulds D, Goa KL: Ticlopidine. *Drugs* 1990; 40:238–259.
7. Meade TW: Low-dose warfarin and low-dose aspirin in the primary prevention of ischemic heart disease. *Am J Cardiol* 1990; 65:7C–11C.
8. Parker JO: Pharmacologic treatment of angina: Nitrate tolerance. *Hosp Pract* 1988; 23(Nov):63–83.
9. Schwartz A: Calcium antagonists: Review and perspective on mechanism of action. *Am J Cardiol* 1989; 64:3I–9I.
10. Scriabine A, Schuurman T, Traber J: Pharmacological basis for the use of nimodipine in central nervous system disorders. *FASEB J* 1989; 3:1799–1806.
11. Sila CA, Furlan AJ: Drug treatment of stroke. *Drugs* 1988; 35:468–476.
12. Uchiyama S, Sone R, Nagayama T, et al: Combination therapy with low-dose aspirin and ticlopidine in cerebral ischemia. *Stroke* 1989; 20:1643–1647.
13. Witztum JL: Current approaches to drug therapy for the hypercholesterolemic patient. *Circulation* 1989; 80:1101–1114.

PART III

Neuropharmacology

Although there has been much research in the areas of neurophysiology and neuropharamacology, we still lack understanding of the complete nature of neurochemicals, such as their sites of release and action and the interactions between neurons. Because of these gaps in our knowledge, pharmacologic treatment of neurologic diseases is not always on a scientific basis. Moreover, chronic use of drugs that affect the central nervous system may cause adaptive changes. The actual mechanisms underlying the therapeutic effect after chronic use may differ from that seen after a single use of the drug.

Neurochemicals can be classified as neurotransmitters, neuromodulators, or neuromediators, depending on whether they have direct or indirect effects on membrane potentials. Neurotransmitters are released from an axon into a synapse, and directly affect membrane potentials. Both the presynaptic and postsynaptic membranes contain receptors for neurochemicals and drugs. Known neurotransmitters include norepinephrine, acetylcholine, dopamine, serotonin, gamma aminobutyric acid, and glycine. A neuromodulator does not directly alter the membrane potential, but affects the ability of neurotransmitters to alter the potential. A neuromediator participates in elicitation of the postsynaptic response to transmitters or modulators.

Neurologic diseases may result from too little or too much of a particular neurochemical in a specific locale. Many neuropharmacologic agents interact with receptors in the nervous system, either as agonists or as antagonists. There are also receptor subtypes in different areas of the brain. Some drugs are more specific for certain receptor subtypes than other drugs. The less specific drugs will obviously have actions in addition to the intended therapeutic action. The drugs are specific for the receptor rather than for the area of the brain. Administration of a drug enables it to bind to its receptors in all areas of the central nervous system, and in the rest of the body, too.

We have made tremendous progress in the past decade in understanding the physiology of mental functions and the pathophysiology of central nervous system disease. This had led to an increase in availability of drugs to treat these specific deficits. Research on humans is difficult, and in many cases there are no appropriate animal models for the specific diseases. Drugs with more specific actions are being developed as our understanding of neurochemistry and specificity of receptors increases.

Correct diagnosis of mental disorders is important in order for appropriate social, psychologic, and pharmacologic treatment to be prescribed. Clinical diagnosis of mental disorders is by criteria established by the American Psychiatric Association and published as *Diagnostic and Statistical Manual of Mental Disorders*, (currently in revised third edition).

This section deals with the psychotropic drugs, those that have an effect on the mental state, such as sedative-hypnotics, antidepressants, and antipsychotics. New federal regulations on use of psychotropic drugs in residents of extended care facilities that participate in Medicare and Medicaid programs will most likely decrease their use. These new laws are in response to studies showing inappropriate diagnosis, dosing regimens, and length of course of treatment.

ADDITIONAL READINGS

1. Cooper JR, Bloom FE, Roth RH: *The Biochemical Basis of Neuropharmacology*, ed 5. New York, Oxford University Press, 1986.
2. *Diagnostic and Statistical Manual of Mental Disorders*, ed 3, revised. Washington, DC, The American Psychiatric Association, 1987.
3. Garrard J, Makris L, Dunham T, et al: Evaluation of neuroleptic drug use by nursing home elderly under proposed Medicare and Medicaid regulations. *JAMA* 1991; 265:463–467.
4. Swonger AK, Constantine LL: *Drugs and Therapy*, ed 2. Boston, Little, Brown & Co, 1983.

Chapter 7

Sedative-Hypnotic Drugs

Sleep disturbances include increased latency in falling asleep, frequent awakenings during the night, and early morning awakening. These are commonly secondary to other problems, such as anxiety, depression, arthritis, and heart failure. In younger adult patients, anxiety and depression are the most common causes of sleep disturbances. In the elderly other medical problems such as pain from musculoskeletal diseases and respiratory distress from heart failure are more often the cause of sleep disturbances. Nonpharmacologic methods of treating sleep problems should be attempted. Changes in before-bedtime habits may be all that are needed. Bedridden people are at risk for nighttime sleep disturbances because of daytime napping. Intermittent napping is likely to cause changes in sleep patterns.

Sedatives decrease neural activity, moderate excitement, calm the patient, produce relaxation, and allow for sleep. Hypnotics produce drowsiness and facilitate onset and maintenance of a state of sleep that resembles natural sleep in electroencephalographic characteristics and from which a person can be easily aroused. However, these drugs can reduce the time spent in rapid eye movement (REM) sleep and can cause a "hangover" effect. Frequently, there is a rebound after the drug is stopped, with nightmares and restlessness occurring. Sedation, hypnosis, and general anesthesia are increasing depths of a continuum of central nervous system depression. Drugs that have a central nervous system depressant action have the potential to have an additive effect on central nervous system depression. These depressants include barbiturates, benzodiazepines, narcotics, and alcohol. Combinations of these agents are potentially lethal.

BARBITURATES

Barbiturates have long been used as sedative-hypnotics. They are used primarily for their hypnotic action, to increase drowsiness, and induce and sustain sleep. There are, however, more efficacious agents for sedation. The benzodiazepines have largely replaced the barbiturates as daytime sedatives, and will be discussed later in

TABLE 7–1.

Correlation of Onset and Duration of Action Times for Barbiturates

Drug Category	Time to Onset	Duration of Action (hr)
Ultrashort acting (anesthetic) Thiopental (Pentothal)	Hypnosis within 30–40 sec, with intravenous administration	0.5
Short acting (sleep inducing) Pentobarbital (Nembutal) Secobarbital (Seconal)	15–30 min	3–6
Intermediate acting (sleep sustaining) Amobarbital (Amytal)	45–60 min	6–10
Long acting (antiepileptic) Phenobarbital (Luminal)	1 hr or more	10–14

this chapter. The barbiturates reversibly depress the activity of all excitable tissue. The central nervous system is particularly sensitive, and depression of its activity is dose dependent—from slight sedation, to surgical anesthesia, to death. At lower doses, the barbiturates are selective for the brain area affected. The reticular activating system is particularly sensitive. The major motor and sensory pathways are not as sensitive. In fact, there may be hyperalgesia. Until the moment of unconsciousness, there is an increased reaction to painful stimuli. Barbiturates cannot produce sedation or sleep in the presence of even moderate pain. In sedative-hypnotic doses, these drugs have little effect on skeletal, cardiac, or smooth muscle excitability. The use of barbiturates as sedative-hypnotics is decreasing. Because of the lack of specificity in their effect on the central nervous system and the possibility of respiratory depression, the barbiturates have a lower therapeutic index than the benzodiazepines. With the barbiturates, tolerance develops more frequently, and there is a greater potential for abuse. The number of drug-drug interactions with barbiturates is high because the barbiturates induce the liver microsomal enzyme system. The use of barbiturates as sedative-hypnotics is also associated with a higher incidence of REM rebound, with an increased incidence of nightmares.

The difference between the various barbiturates is their duration of action, from ultrashort to long acting (Table 7–1). The duration of action correlates with the time to onset of action. The long-acting barbiturate phenobarbital (Luminal) has a latency of an hour or more and a duration of action of 10 to 14 hours. This drug is used for its antiepileptic properties. The intermediate acting agent amobarbital (Amytal) is used as a sleep sustainer. It has a latency of 45 to 60 minutes and a duration of action of 6 to 10 hours. The short acting barbiturates, pentobarbital (Nembutal) and secobarbital (Seconal), are used as sleep inducers. They have a latency of 15 to 30 minutes and a duration of 3 to 6 hours. For hypnotic use, the drugs are administered before bedtime at a dose of 100 mg for pentobarbital and 50 to 200 mg for secobarbital. The ultrashort acting barbiturate, thiopental (Pentothal) is used as an intravenous anesthetic.

The effects of barbiturates on sleep are different when first used by a patient compared with chronic use. With first use or occasional use, and for one night only, there is suppression of REM sleep. On the next night, without the drug, there is increased time spent in REM sleep, so-called REM rebound. With chronic use, tolerance to REM suppression develops over 1 to 2 weeks, so the time spent in REM sleep returns to normal. With withdrawal after chronic use, there is an increased percent of time spent in REM sleep, although the total sleep time decreases during the withdrawal period.

The barbiturates are metabolized in the liver by the microsomal enzyme system. This class of drugs also induces the activity of this enzyme system. The enzyme induction is responsible for metabolic tolerance to the barbiturates and for many drug interactions with the barbiturates (see the section "Tolerance" later in this chapter).

Adverse effects

Adverse effects from barbiturate use are dose related and are mostly an extension of their actions. Severe intoxication causes general nervous system depression, including depression of the respiratory center in the medulla oblongata. Respiratory center depression is frequently the cause of death in cases of barbiturate overdose. The residual depression or hangover observed with barbiturate use relates to the duration of action of the agent. This effect is noticed less with the short acting than with the intermediate or long acting agents.

Tolerance

Tolerance, both functional and metabolic, develops to the barbiturates; however, the functional tolerance is more important and occurs faster. Functional tolerance refers to the adjustment of the brain neurochemistry to the continuous presence of a drug in such a manner that the same dose of the drug becomes less capable of modifying brain function. In other words, it takes more and more of the drug to produce the same effect. As tolerance increases, the therapeutic index, toxic dose/effective dose, decreases because tolerance affects only the effective dose but has little or no effect on toxicity. Cross-tolerance to all central nervous system depressants—alcohol, benzodiazepines, and narcotics—develops. All can maintain dependence for each other, and postpone the onset of withdrawal symptoms.

The metabolic tolerance is due to enhancement of the mircosomal enzyme system of the liver by barbiturates. Tolerance occurs because of rapid inactivation of the drug, with decreased duration of action and decreased intensity of action of drugs metabolized by this system. Other drugs metabolized by this enzyme system are warfarin (Coumadin), digitoxin, propranolol (Inderal), quinidine, phenytoin (Dilantin), and the tricyclic antidepressants. Also, steroid hormones are metabolized by this enzyme system. A serious problem can occur if a person is taking a barbiturate and then warfarin is administered. Warfarin would be titrated to its therapeutic effect. Because of the increased metabolism of warfarin, the dose of warfarin needed will be higher than in the nonbarbiturate user. If the barbiturate were then suddenly stopped, the warfarin dose would be too high and would be likely to cause serious hemorrhage.

Chronic overuse

Chronic overuse produces a sequence of personality changes related to affectual or mood effects of the drugs. The early effects may be euphoria or depression. With depression there may be an increase in suicidal tendencies. Drugs that depress the central nervous system can worsen depressive symptoms. With progressive use, affectual changes can lead to emotional lability, characterized by lack of motivation, slovenliness, and confusion. Hallucinations may occur in chronic intoxication, and occasionally chronic psychoses will develop. Neurologic manifestations of barbiturate intoxication include slurring of speech, double vision, vertigo, and difficulties of visual accommodation and gait.

Withdrawal

After chronic use of a barbiturate, abrupt discontinuance of the drug causes "withdrawal" symptoms. The severity of the withdrawal reaction is related to the intensity of the addiction. Withdrawal from barbiturate addiction produces symptoms similar to those seen upon alcohol withdrawal. Depending on the severity, the following may be seen or experienced: anxiety, insomnia, muscle twitches, tremors, weakness, nausea, vomiting, illusions and delusions, hallucinations and paranoia, delirium, convulsive seizures, and death.

BENZODIAZEPINES

The benzodiazepines are one of the more frequently prescribed classes of drugs. The central nervous system effects of the benzodiazepines are sedation, hypnosis, decreased anxiety, and muscle relaxation. Some drugs in this class are used for their anticonvulsant properties. (Their use other than for sedation-hypnosis will be discussed in the appropriate sections.) The benzodiazepines are not general neuronal depressants, as are the barbiturates. They do not cause surgical anesthesia. They act on the limbic system and spinal cord, but do not significantly depress the cerebral cortex. Their actions are a result of potentiation of the neural inhibition mediated by gamma aminobutyric acid (GABA). Their effects on the respiratory and cardiovascular systems are minor. Overall, the benzodiazepines have a larger margin of safety than the barbiturates. They do not depress REM sleep. However, suddenly stopping the drug after chronic use can lead to withdrawal symptoms, including insomnia and anxiety. The drug dose should be slowly reduced over a period of time to prevent withdrawal symptoms from occurring. Slowly withdrawing a drug after chronic use is called "tapering".

Of the benzodiazepines, only three are currently approved for use as hypnotics:

TABLE 7–2.

Benzodiazepines

Drug	Half-life (hr)	Dose Range (mg)
Triazolam (Halcion)	2–5	0.125–0.25
Temazepam (Restoril)	10	15–30
Flurazepam (Dalmane)	47–100	15–30

flurazepam (Dalmane), temazepam (Restoril), and triazolam (Halcion) (Table 7–2). These are useful for short-term treatment of insomnia, for no longer than a few weeks. The major problem with the use of benzodiazepines as sedative-hypnotics is the possibility of residual daytime sedation. Sedation and ataxia increase the risk of falls and fractures, especially in the elderly. This may occur even with doses within the recommended therapeutic range.

Flurazepam (Dalmane) has a rapid onset of action of 30 to 60 minutes, and, with an elimination half-life of 47 to 100 hours, has the potential to accumulate in the body with daily use. This can lead to residual daytime sedation and impaired cognitive and psychomotor function. In the elderly, the risk of falls and fractures increases with the use of the longer acting drugs. Flurazepam is the only hypnotic with effectiveness beyond 2 weeks of nightly use. It apparently has a lesser abuse potential than the others. It also has excellent skeletal muscle relaxant properties.

Temazepam (Restoril), with a mean half-life of 10 hours, and triazolam (Halcion), with a half-life of about 2 to 5 hours, have less potential for residual sedation. Temazepam has an onset of action of 1 to 2 hours but, with its longer half-life, is effective throughout the sleeping time and may be more effective for those people who have problems with staying asleep and with early morning awakening. Triazolam has an onset of action of 30 to 60 minutes, and with its short half-life, may be preferable for those people who only have problems falling asleep. Triazolam, however, has been associated with short-term memory loss and may be responsible for rebound insomnia, especially after long-term use. Tapering the dose after chronic use is recommended to prevent these problems.

The benzodiazepines are metabolized in the liver, sometimes to other active products. The half-lives listed reflect all biologically active metabolites. They are highly bound to plasma proteins, but this is apparently of no clinical significance. There do not seem to be any drug interactions at this level. These drugs do not induce the liver drug metabolizing enzymes. However, aging and liver disease can affect metabolism of these drugs. With decreased metabolism and elimination of the drugs, the half-life, and thus the duration of action, is increased.

Adverse effects

Adverse effects from the benzodiazepines are drowsiness, lethargy, mental confusion, and impairment of mental and psychomotor function. These effects are more likely in the elderly and are related to dosage and duration of action. The higher the dose and the longer the elimination half-life, the greater are the chances for adverse effects. In the elderly, the risk of falling increases with psychotropic drug use. Thus, the lower end of the dose range is more appropriate in elderly patients.

OTHERS

Over-the-counter sleep-inducing drugs are used by many people. An antihistamine, either diphenhydramine or doxylamine, is the active ingredient. Their effectiveness as sedatives-hypnotics, although variable, is attributed to the drowsiness side effect of the antihistimines. Development of tolerance and inadequacy of dosage contribute to the lack of effectiveness. There is also the possibility of residual daytime sedation. Over-the-counter drugs that contain diphenhydramine are Sominex, Nytol, Compoz, Sleep-Eze 3, and Sleepinal. Unisom contains doxylamine, which is another antihistamine with central nervous system actions. The central nervous system depressant action of the antihistimines is additive to that of other depressants.

PHYSICAL THERAPY NOTES

Daytime sedation resulting from sedative-hypnotic use can significantly impair physical therapy treatment. Mental alertness may be decreased and may affect the patient's ability to concentrate and to follow instructions. The patient may appear confused and uncooperative. Attention span and memory may be affected by some of these drugs. Functional ability also may be reduced. There may be associated personality changes, ranging from euphoria, to depression, to apathy. Patients may experience dizziness and vertigo on arising, with an increased risk of injuries from falls. The patient needs to be instructed to arise slowly, to the sitting position, and then to standing. Ambulation assistance may be needed. The risk of falling increases with residual sedative effects. Guarding against falls and subsequent fractures is important, especially with the elderly. A fear of falling may develop in a person who has experienced recurrent dizziness and vertigo, leading to a feeling of frustration and dependency. Deviations in gait may become evident.

Over-the-counter drugs containing antihistamines can cause sedation, and this can be a particular problem in the elderly. Multidrug cold capsules are likely to contain antihistamines.

LEARNING OBJECTIVES

1. Understand the difference between sedation and hypnosis.
2. List the classes of drugs used to treat insomnia.

3. Understand the mechanisms of drug tolerance in relation to barbiturate use.
4. Describe untoward effects on patients with use of the sedative-hypnotics and how these may interfere with physical therapy treatment.
5. Understand the influence of sedative-hypnotics on sleep patterns, both with acute and chronic administration.

ADDITIONAL READINGS

1. Ho IK: Mechanism of action of barbiturates. *Annu Rev Pharmacol Toxicol* 1981; 21:83–111.
2. Kales A, Kales JD, Soldatos CR: Insomnia and other sleep disorders. *Med Clin North Am* 1982; 66:971–991.
3. Moran MG, Thompson TL, Nies AS: Sleep disorders in the elderly. *Am J Psychiatry* 1988; 145:1369–1378.
4. Nicholson AN: The use of short- and long-acting hypnotics in clinical medicine. *Br J Clin Pharmacol* 1981; 11:61S–69S.

Chapter 8

Antianxiety Drugs

Anxiety is described as a feeling of heightened tension, apprehensiveness, or uneasiness. Everyone has experienced anxiety at one time or another. It can range from "butterflies in the stomach" with tachycardia to the more debilitating panic disorders and phobias that interfere with normal function. The normal anxieties associated with everyday living are not treated with antianxiety drugs. A little anxiety may help a person confront a new or stressful situation, for example, a major test in school or a new job. Generally, acute episodes of anxiety resolve spontaneously. Only when anxiety becomes incapacitating is pharmacologic treatment necessary. Symptoms of anxiety are frequently related to stimulation of the autonomic nervous system, with tachycardia and palpitations, motor tension, and apprehension. Also, dyspnea, a choking or smothering sensation, and a feeling of not being in control are frequently experienced. Classes of clinical anxiety include panic attacks, generalized anxiety disorder, and the obsessive-compulsive disorder (OCD). Panic attacks are discreet periods of intense feelings with a sudden onset. These attacks usually last minutes, but may occur for longer periods of time. Generalized anxiety disorder is characterized by excessive apprehension or fear, unrealistic for the situation, lasting for 6 months or longer. Obsessive-compulsive disorder is characterized by the existence of obsessions and/or compulsions that are either time consuming or interfere with occupational and social functioning. Only when one cannot cope with or dissipate the anxiety does it become maladaptive. Anxiety is one of the most commonly treated mental disorders. Drugs that are used to treat anxieties are called antianxiety agents of anxiolytics. They have formerly been referred to as minor tranquilizers, as opposed to the antipsychotic drugs, the major tranquilizers.

Depression is frequently encountered with anxiety disorders, and both often accompany underlying medical diseases. It is thought by some that anxiety and depression may be part of the same behavioral disorder, with different manifestations—anxiety or depression—at different times. This section discusses the treatment of anxiety itself. The next chapter covers the treatment of depression.

The underlying biochemical abnormality in anxiety is not known. However, research into the actions of agents that are effective in treating anxiety disorders has given us some information on the neurochemical imbalance. The benzodiazepines, which have actions additional to their anxiolytic effects, potentiate the neural inhibition mediated by gamma aminobutyric acid (GABA). Some newer agents, which are more selective anxiolytics, act through the serotonin system. Buspirone (Buspar) is an effective anxiolytic, which acts to increase the action of serotonin. This agent, rather than inhibiting reuptake, acts as a serotonin receptor agonist. There are, however, several serotonin receptor subtypes. Further research is needed to understand the operation of these different receptor types. The efficacy of buspirone in OCD supports the role of serotonin in this disorder.

BENZODIAZEPINES

The anxiolytic action of the benzodiazepines may result from actions in the limbic system and reticular formation. These drugs do not significantly depress the cerebral cortex. Central nervous system effects of the benzodiazepines are sedation, hypnosis, decreased anxiety, and muscle relaxation. Some benzodiazepines are used for their anticonvulsant properties and are discussed in Chapter 12, Antiepileptics. The benzodiazepines are not general neuronal depressants and do not cause surgical anesthesia, like the barbiturates. They produce sedation, but have a flatter dose-response curve in producing a mild sedation compared with the barbiturates. They act on the limbic system and spinal cord, but do not significantly depress the cerebral cortex. The actions are a result of potentiation of the neural inhibition mediated by GABA. Their effects on the respiratory and cardiovascular systems are minor. They reduce the level of central nervous system excitability and inhibit the physiologic changes produced by anxiety. The trembling, sweating, nausea, increased rate of respiration, increased heart rate, and increased blood pressure, are eliminated or reduced in intensity.

Diazepam (Valium) is the most commonly used of the benzodiazepines. They are all about equally effective as anxiolytics, but the side effects vary. The benzodiazepines with the shorter half-lives, lorazepam (Ativan), oxazepam (Serax), and alprazolam (Xanax), produce less daytime sedation. Chlordiazepoxide (Librium) is more sedative than diazepam. The benzodiazepines that are used as anxiolytics are listed in Table 8–1.

Adverse effects

Adverse effects of the benzodiazepines, and signs of excess central nervous system depression, are drowsiness, lethargy, mental confusion, ataxia, and disorientation. These are more likely in the elderly. The potential for abuse and dependence with these drugs is variable. Addiction can occur, but usually results from excessive doses or a prolonged duration of treatment, longer than 2 months. There are problems with long-term use, especially at the higher doses and in combination with

TABLE 8–1.

Anxiolytics

Drug	Half-life (hr)	Daily Dose Range (adult) (mg)
Benzodiazepines		
Diazepam (Valium)	30–60	2–40
Chlordiazepoxide (Librium)	28–48	10–80
Oxazepam (Serax)	6–11	30–120
Clorazepate (Tranxene)	50–80	15–60
Lorazepam (Ativan)	12–15	1–10
Alprazolam (Xanax)	12–15	0.5–4
Prazepam (Centrax)	40–70	20–60
Other anxiolytics		
Meprobamate (Miltown)	6–17	1,200–1,600
Hydroxyzine (Atarax, Vistaril)	3	200–400
Buspirone (Buspar)	2–3	20–30

other abused drugs. Suddenly stopping the drug after chronic use can cause withdrawal symptoms. Withdrawal symptoms, especially rebound agitation and insomnia, may be seen in about half the people taking these drugs, and symptoms may persist for months. Gradual withdrawal is recommended to reduce the incidence and severity of withdrawal symptoms. In spite of these potential hazards, benzodiazepines are considered relatively safe, and they are rarely fatal by themselves. True coma is uncommon. One rarely sees respiratory or cardiovascular depression except in chronic obstructive pulmonary disease, when respiration may be compromised. The long-acting benzodiazepines have a more prolonged half-life in the elderly. This can cause central nervous system toxicity, such as confusion and oversedation, that can lead to falls and the possibility of fractures. The benzodiazepines are additive with other depressants, such as alcohol, barbiturates, and opiate narcotics, in central nervous system depression.

OTHER ANXIOLYTICS

Meprobamate (Miltown, Equanil) is an effective skeletal muscle relaxant; however, tolerance develops with continued use. Also, it has a higher reported incidence of dependence, and withdrawal symptoms are common after long-term use. Drowsiness is a frequent side effect, with ataxia evident at high doses. Hypotension is seen frequently in those taking this drug.

Hydroxyzine (Atarax, Vistaril) is an antihistamine with sedative and antianxiety properties. The adult dose is 200 to 400 mg/day, taken in divided doses. It has a rapid onset of action, with clinical effects seen 15 to 30 minutes after oral administration. Side effects are minimal and may be limited to the anticholinergic-induced dry mouth. Additive central nervous system depression is seen with other depressants, such as barbiturates and alcohol.

Buspirone (Buspar) is a selective anxiolytic agent. It is a serotonin receptor agonist, but the relationship of serotonin to its antianxiety action is unknown. There is no cross-tolerance to other central nervous system depressants, such as alcohol, barbiturates, or benzodiazepines and it does not provide relief from withdrawal symptoms of the sedatives discussed earlier. It is not a muscle relaxant, nor is it anticonvulsive. There is no evidence that it causes physical dependence. It has minimal potential for abuse and addiction. There is also a lack of withdrawal symptoms on discontinuance of the drug. Buspirone also causes less sedation than the benzodiazepines and causes less impairment of motor performance.

Buspirone is bound to plasma proteins, but this does not appear to cause problems with displacement of other drugs from plasma proteins. It is metabolized in the liver, and the metabolites are excreted mainly by the kidney. The plasma elimination half-life is 2 to 3 hours. The recommended daily dose is 20 to 30 mg, taken in divided doses. It has limited side effects as far as causing drowsiness or reducing functional ability. It can be used in combination with other psychotropics, except the antipsychotic monoamine oxidase inhibitors and haloperidol (Haldol). The pharmacokinetics are similar in the elderly as in younger people. With the new federal regulations restricting use of psychotropic drugs in long-term care facilities, the use of nonsedating anxiolytics such as buspirone may increase.

PHYSICAL THERAPY NOTES

Although daytime sedation is not so much a problem with the benzodiazepines as with the barbiturates, overdosage can cause oversedation and ataxia. Sedating drugs have the potential to impair motor or cognitive functioning. Therefore, all precautions mentioned in Chapter 7 for the sedative-hypnotics regarding the effects these impairments have on physical therapy treatment also apply here.

Anxiety, especially in a new situation, is common and is considered a normal behavioral response. Many patients experience some degree of apprehension on their first visit to physical therapy. This may relate to their uncertainties concerning their present condition. The behavioral aspect of physical therapy treatment is very important in relieving minor anxiety, which will optimize any treatment given.

LEARNING OBJECTIVES

1. Understand the differences between barbiturates and benzodiazepines, especially as they relate to the problem of daytime sedation.
2. Describe the effects of overdosage of the benzodiazepines and relate these to interference with physical therapy treatment.

ADDITIONAL READINGS

1. Dominguez RA: The benzodiazepines: A current review for the nonpsychiatrist. *Hosp Formul* 1983; 18:1049–1056.
2. Meyer BR: Benzodiazepines in the elderly. *Med Clin North Am* 1982; 66:1017–1035.
3. Stavrakaki C, Vargo B: The relationship of anxiety and depression: A review of the literature. *Br J Psychiatry* 1986; 149:7–16.
4. Taylor DP: Buspirone, a new approach to the treatment of anxiety. *FASEB J* 1988; 2:2445–2452.
5. Woods JH, Katz JL, Winger G: Abuse liability of benzodiazepines. *Pharmacol Rev* 1987; 39: 251–413.

Chapter 9

Drugs Used in Treatment of Mood Disorders

Most people experience variations in mood, even within a day. Depression may be a normal functional process, such as grief following loss of a loved one. Secondary contributing factors are other medical conditions and side effects from certain drugs. Medical conditions that can cause complaints of fatigue and weakness (which also are associated with depression) are anemia, hypoglycemia, hypokalemia, Cushing's syndrome, and heart failure. Drugs that can cause depression as a side effect are beta blockers, methyldopa (Aldomet), glucocorticoids, cimetidine (Tagemet), and the benzodiazepines. The clinical diagnosis of depression or mania is based on both the duration and the intensity of the mood alteration. Many psychiatrists think that mood is a continuum, from depression to mania. When a person's mood is at either end of the spectrum, then it may interfere with appropriate social and occupational function.

Mood disorders, also called affective disorders, include depressive disorders and bipolar disorders. Depressive disorders are characterized by one or more periods of depression without manic or hypomanic episodes. The essential feature of bipolar disorders is one or more manic or hypomanic episodes, usually accompanied by one or more major depressive episodes.

A major depressive episode is defined as a depressed mood or loss of interest or pleasure in all or almost all activities for at least a 2-week duration. Accompanying symptoms of depression are many and all may not be present in each depressive episode. A person may experience a change in appetite—generally decreased but it may be increased—resulting in a corresponding change in weight. Sleep disturbances may manifest as either insomnia or hypersomnia. There is frequently a decrease in energy and a withdrawal from family and friends associated with lack of interest in previously pleasurable activities. Feelings of worthlessness and guilt, along with recurrent thoughts of death and suicidal thoughts and attempts, are often accompanying symptoms. During a depressive episode a person has difficulty in concentrating and is easily distracted.

The essential feature of a manic episode is a distinct period during which the predominant mood is either elevated, expansive, or irritable. It may be sufficiently severe to cause marked impairment in occupational function or in usual social activities or relationships, or even to require hospitalization to prevent harm to the person or to others. The person has an inflated self esteem or feelings of grandiosity, a decreased need for sleep, and is easily distracted. The elevated mood is described as not only euphoric, but also excessive. In hypomania the symptoms are less severe and delusions are not present. The impairment is generally not sufficiently severe to require hospitalization.

Mood disorders have a genetic component, which is highly influenced by the environment. Genetic vulnerability can make a person more sensitive to environmental insults. However, it is not possible to predict that a particular major external event, for example, the death of a child, will cause a depressive episode in a person. The genetic aspect of depression is thought to be related to a deficiency of one or more of the neurotransmitters in crucial areas of the brain. Most currently available antidepressant drugs appear to interfere with the metabolism or reuptake of one or more of the neurotransmitters and thus may act to increase the concentration of the neurotransmitter in the synapse. At variance with this neurotransmitter deficiency theory is the fact that blockade of neurotransmitter uptake occurs within hours, whereas clinical efficacy of the antidepressants take weeks to occur. Nevertheless, the antidepressants are grouped according to their major action on neurotransmitter metabolism. Many older reuptake inhibitors have actions on more than one transmitter. The newer agents are more selective and generally block reuptake of a single neurotransmitter. This avoids the common side effects of the antidepressants. The tricyclic drugs are likely to have anticholinergic and cardiovascular side effects. The monoamine oxidase inhibitors are more likely to cause postural hypotension; however, dietary and drug interactions carry the risk of hypertensive crisis.

Depression is a common mood disorder of the elderly. Depression can be brought on or intensified by diabetes mellitus, metabolic disorders, thyroid disease, severe anemia, mononucleosis, hypertension, and cancer. Also depressant drugs, such as alcohol, antihistamines, anticholinergics, barbiturates, and the benzodiazepines, can cause depression. Depression resulting from a metabolic or toxic cause is best treated by removal of the precipitating factor rather than by use of the antidepressants.

MONOAMINE OXIDASE INHIBITORS

Drugs in this class inhibit the monoamine oxidase enzyme in the nerve terminals. This enzyme is responsible for metabolism of norepinephrine. Thus, enzyme inhibition increases the level of norepinephrine in the synapse, which is then available to interact with receptors. Two to 4 weeks of treatment are required before a therapeutic effect is seen. The monoamine oxidase inhibitors currently in use are

TABLE 9–1.

Monoamine Oxidase Inhibitors

Drug	Total Daily Dose (mg)
Tranylcypromine (Parnate)	10–30
Isocarboxazid (Marplan)	10–30
Phenelzine sulfate (Nardil)	60–90

listed in Table 9–1. These drugs are readily absorbed after oral administration. Therapeutic effectiveness is maintained by once a day treatment.

The increased sympathetic nervous system activity is usually associated with a decreased parasympathetic nervous system activity, with dry mouth, dizziness, constipation, urinary difficulties, delayed ejaculation, and impotence. A potentially serious problem with the use of monoamine oxidase inhibitors (MAOIs) is that, in combination with tyramine in certain foods, they can cause a hypertensive crisis. Tyramine in these foods acts indirectly, by displacing norepinephrine from nerve terminals to the extracellular fluid. Those people taking MAOIs should avoid foods and beverages containing tyramines, such as aged cheeses (e.g., cheddar, old center cut, aged in alcohol, Camembert, Stilton, or Gruyere), pickled herring, salted dry herring, chicken livers, pods of broad beans, Chianti wine, some beers, and yeast extracts.

Side effects are the possibility of orthostatic hypotension. This may require a reduction in dose. The MAOIs can cause liver damage, but this is rarely a problem at the doses normally employed.

TRICYCLIC ANTIDEPRESSANTS

This class of drugs is so named because of the chemical structure. These agents have no stimulatory effect in healthy individuals; in fact, they produce mostly unpleasant feelings. However, when administered to clinically depressed patients, the drugs cause an elevation of mood. Clinical improvement in mood may take 2 to 3 weeks of treatment, and the full therapeutic effect may not be seen until 4 weeks of treatment. Their mechanism of action is thought to relate to prevention of norepinephrine reuptake by the presynaptic nerve terminals. In spite of the long time required for clinical improvement, norepinephrine reuptake blockade is established promptly. The tricyclic antidepressants are listed in Table 9–2. The tricyclics are well absorbed from the gastrointestinal tract after oral administration. They are metabolized in the liver, some to other active products. In children and in adults over 60 years of age they are metabolized more slowly. With the tricyclics there is a wide variability in dosage requirements because of individual differences in absorption and metabolism.

Clomipramine (Anafranil), although structurally a tricyclic, is a selective seroto-

TABLE 9–2.

Tricyclic Antidepressants

Drug	Total Daily Dose (mg)
Amitriptyline (Elavil, Endep)	50–150
Desipramine (Norpramin)	100–300
Doxepin (Adapin, Sinequan)	75–150
Imipramine (Tofranil)	30–200
Nortriptyline (Aventyl, Pamelor)	75–100
Protriptyline (Vivactil)	15–60
Clomipramine (Anafranil)	100–250
Amoxapine (Asendin)	200–300
Trimipramine (Surmontil)	50–150
Maprotiline (Ludiomil)	50–150

nin reuptake inhibitor. It is used therapeutically in treatment of obsessive-compulsive disorder (OCD). Maprotiline (Ludiomil) is structurally a tetracyclic; however, it has a pharmacologic profile similar to tricyclics, so it is included with this class of antidepressants.

ATYPICAL ANTIDEPRESSANTS

The atypical antidepressants (Table 9–3) constitute a new generation of effective antidepressants, generally lacking the central and peripheral anticholinergic, cardiovascular, and sedative properties of the tricyclics. The neurotransmitters more selectively affected by these drugs are serotonin and dopamine. These drugs may be safer in patients with cardiovascular disease.

Fluoxetine (Prozac) has recently been introduced to the U.S. market. It has a more selective action to inhibit serotonin uptake. Its adverse effects are nervousness/anxiety, insomnia, gastrointestinal disturbances of nausea and diarrhea, and headache. It has an anorexic effect with weight loss, opposite to the tricyclics. Its stimulatory, rather than sedating, effect limits its usefulness in panic disorders. In fact, this drug may lead to mania. Fluoxetine has been charged with causing violent suicidal preoccupation in some patients. However, untreated depressed patients also have suicidal tendencies.

Trazodone (Desyrel) also has antiserotonin as well as serotoninergic actions. Opposed to fluoxetine, trazodone is sedating. However, like fluoxetine, it is without anticholinergic actions and has fewer cardiac effects than the tricyclics.

Buspirone (Buspar) acts as a serotonin agonist, rather than as a reuptake inhibitor. It has been mentioned in Chapter 8 as an anxiolytic. The anxiolytic and antidepressant actions are dose dependent, with anxiolytic actions seen at lower doses (20 to 30 mg/day) and antidepressant actions at higher doses (40 to 50 mg/day). Side effects that may be encountered with buspirone (Buspar) are headache, dizziness,

TABLE 9–3.

Atypical Antidepressants

Drug	Total Daily Dose (mg)
Serotonin reuptake inhibitors	
Fluoxetine (Prozac)	20–80
Trazodone (Desyrel)	150–400
Buspirone (Buspar)	40–50
Dopamine reuptake inhibitors	
Bupropion (Wellbutrin)	200–300

and nausea. It, however, has no effect on appetite and it has no anticholinergic side effects. The effectiveness of fluoxetine and buspirone in anxiety and depression lends support to the theory that serotonin is involved in these disorders and that they may be a part of the same disorder.

Both buspirone and fluoxetine are effective in treatment of OCD, as well as clomipramine (see Tricyclic Antidepressants, earlier in this chapter). Obsessive-compulsive disorder is classified as an anxiety disorder and is characterized by the existence of obsessions and/or compulsions that are time consuming or interfere with occupational and social functioning. The action of these drugs on the serotonin system suggests a role for serotonin in this disorder also.

Bupropion (Wellbutrin) is a dopamine reuptake inhibitor that has little anticholinergic activity and causes neither Electrocardiographic (EKG) changes nor orthostatic hypotension. This agent is not sedating and does not stimulate appetite; in fact, it often depresses appetite and leads to a decrease in body weight.

Adverse effects of tricyclic and atypical antidepressants

Efficacy does not vary much among the different tricyclics; however, there is a wide variability in side effects. The tricyclics can cause a direct depression of the myocardium. This is potentially dangerous if preexisting conduction defects exist, especially bundle branch block. These drugs also have anticholinergic and anti–alpha adrenergic actions, which may result in tachycardia, cardiac arrhythmias, and orthostatic hypotension. Amitriptyline (Elavil) and imipramine (Tofranil) can cause EKG changes, worsen heart failure, and provoke atrial and ventricular arrhythmias. However, under some circumstances, these agents may be antiarrhythmic. Their use in the elderly is a dilemma, as depression is common in this age group, which is also more likely to show cardiac problems. Postural hypotension is a common side effect of the cyclics and can be serious. Amoxapine (Asendin), desipramine (Norpramin), and nortriptyline (Aventyl, Pamelor) are less likely to produce postural hypotension than the other tricyclics. The atypical antidepressants, fluoxetine and trazodone, also are less likely to have cardiac effects.

Anticholinergic symptoms result from blockade of acetylcholine. Dry mouth, constipation, blurred vision, and urinary retention are the most common among the older drugs amitriptyline, imipramine, trimipramine, nortriptyline, and doxepin. These side effects may be only uncomfortable in younger patients; however, in elderly or medically compromised patients, they may be hazardous. These particular drugs are also more likely to cause confusion, memory impairment, and stuttering speech. In the elderly, concurrent use of other drugs that have anticholinergic effects, such as antihistamines and anticholinergics used in treatment of Parkinson's disease, can lead to serious mental confusion. Of the tricyclics, amitriptyline is the most anticholinergic and causes sedation. The anticholinergic activity of the tricyclics in descending order, from most anticholinergic to least, is amitriptyline > doxepin > imipramine = protriptyline > nortriptyline = desipramine. Amitriptyline and doxepin, being sedatives, may help in those patients with insomnia and agitation. Desipramine, which is not sedative, may in fact worsen insomnia. Urinary retention is more of a problem in elderly men, especially those with prostatic hypertrophy. The atypical antidepressants have less anticholinergic effects.

Most of the tricyclics have an appetite stimulating effect, which may lead to weight gain if nutrition is not monitored properly. Desipramine, amoxapine, and trazadone are less likely than other tricyclics to increase appetite.

Some of the antidepressant drugs can provoke seizures, especially with higher doses, and in those patients with a history of convulsive disorders. Maprotiline (Ludiomil) and bupropion (Wellbutrin) are more likely to produce seizures, especially at higher doses.

Tricyclics have the potential to interact with the antihypertensive drugs clonidine (Catapres), methyldopa (Aldomet), propranolol (Inderal), and metoprolol (Lopressor). The antihypertensives interfere with the action of the tricyclics, and the tricyclics block the action of the antihypertensives that act on central alpha receptors.

In the elderly and in adolescents, it is generally best to start with a low dose and gradually increase the dose, if necessary. These age groups are especially sensitive to adverse effects of the tricyclics. A single daily dose in the evening is usually effective and minimizes anticholinergic effects, which may be more bothersome during the day. Also, lower doses are recommended for outpatients where direct medical supervision is not possible.

Acute poisoning is a serious risk for those people with suicidal tendencies. The central nervous system depressant actions of alcohol and other sedatives are potentiated by the antidepressants. Overdose from antidepressants is a common cause of drug-related deaths.

LITHIUM

Lithium carbonate (Eskalith, Lithane) has a mood-stabilizing effect on patients with manic-depressive illness, particularly during the manic phase. This agent may be used along with the tricyclic antidepressants in treatment of bipolar disorders. Lithium affects neurotransmitter systems in a variety of ways, but no one known mechanism of action accounts for its clinical effects.

Lithium is well absorbed from the gastrointestinal tract after oral administration and is excreted almost entirely by the kidney. It has an elimination half-life of about 24 hours, with increases seen with aging, as kidney function decreases. Decreased kidney function is a contraindication to lithium use. About 7 to 10 days of treatment are usually required before a full therapeutic effect is seen.

Side effects are seen at initiation of treatment as gastrointestinal irritation with epigastric discomfort, fine hand tremor, fatigue, and drowsiness. Toxicity of higher levels of lithium is seen as nausea, diarrhea, vomiting, significant hand tremor, cogwheel rigidity, aphasia, and delirium. One of the first signs of toxicity is an increase in deep tendon reflexes and muscle fasciculations. Plasma concentrations can be monitored along with clinical status in an effort to maintain effective dosage and to avoid toxicity. Lithium is teratogenic and should be avoided in pregnancy, especially during the first trimester. Lithium generally should not be administered to those people taking diuretics. Diuretics decrease renal clearance of lithium and increase the risk of lithium toxicity.

Other agents with antimanic actions are the antiepileptics carbamazepine (Tegretol) and valproic acid (Depakene). Although there is not a lot of experience to date with these drugs in treatment of bipolar illness, they may be of particular use in those people who do not respond to lithium.

PHYSICAL THERAPY NOTES

The most common complaints associated with depression are lack of energy and motivation, fatigue, and gastrointestinal symptoms. Depressive symptoms can interfere with physical therapy treatment. If the patient is sufficiently withdrawn, the lack of interest in therapy and the lack of motivation will interfere with treatment. Many ill people are depressed as a normal reaction to their clinical situation. The behavioral aspect of physical therapy is important in alleviating this type of temporary depression. Exercise, diet, and social environment can be supportive measures.

Adverse effects of drugs used in treatment of mood disorders can interfere with physical therapy treatment. The possibility of postural hypotension as a side effect from the monoamine oxidase inhibitors and the cyclics should be of concern to physical therapists. The danger from falls and subsequent fractures has been mentioned. For a more complete discussion of postural hypotension, see Chapter 21. The tricyclic antidepressants pose a potential risk to certain cardiac patients, especially in regard to arrhythmias. Amoxapine (Asendin) can cause extrapyramidal symptoms. This drug also has the possibility of leading to tardive dyskinesia. Central anticholinergic actions of the tricyclic drugs can lead to mental confusion. Their antihistamine actions can lead to drowsiness.

In patients treated with lithium, the lithium levels are monitored in order to prevent toxicity. However, clinical signs and symptoms are also important. Increased deep tendon reflexes, hand tremor, fatigue, drowsiness, and slurred speech are easily noted by the physical therapist.

Depression can appear as a side effect to a drug. Clonidine (Catapres), hydralazine (Apresoline), and other central nervous system depressants, can cause depression.

LEARNING OBJECTIVES

1. Understand the proposed mechanisms of action of the antidepressants as related to neurotransmitters.
2. Know the side effects of the drugs that relate to an extension of the pharmacologic effects, for example, the anticholinergic actions of the tricyclics.
3. Describe the side effects of the various drugs that would have an impact on physical therapy treatment, for example, postural hypotension, extrapyramidal symptoms.
4. Describe the interaction of certain foods with monoamine oxidase inhibitors.
5. List the side effects of lithium toxicity.

ADDITIONAL READINGS

1. Coryell W, Keller M, Lavori P, et al: Affective syndromes, psychotic features, and prognosis. I: Depression. *Arch Gen Psychiatry* 1990; 47:651–657.
2. Coryell W, Keller M, Lavori P, et al: Affective syndromes, psychotic features, and prognosis. II: Mania. *Arch Gen Psychiatry* 1990; 47:658–662.
3. Furlanut M, Benetello P: The pharmacokinetics of tricyclic antidepressant drugs in the elderly. *Pharmacol Res* 1990; 22:15–25.
4. Rudorfer MV, Potter WZ: Antidepressants. *Drugs* 1989; 37:713–738.
5. Shaw DM: Drug alternatives to lithium in manic-depressive disorders. *Drugs* 1988; 36:249–255.

Chapter 10

Antipsychotic Drugs

The psychoses are conditions in which the mental functioning of an individual is sufficiently impaired to interfere with ordinary demands of life. There is decreased acceptance of reality and an inability to appropriately function in one's current environment. The major psychoses are schizophrenia, delusional disorders, some organic mental diseases, and some mood disorders. Complete treatment of psychotic patients requires more than pharmacotherapy. Psychologic and other supportive measures are necessary for complete rehabilitation of the psychotic patient.

Schizophrenia is a psychotic disorder characterized by disturbances in affect and development of thought, and includes the presence of delusions and hallucinations. The criteria for diagnosis of schizophrenia are listed in Table 10–1. The mental function is sufficiently impaired to interfere with ordinary demands of social and occupational functions. Schizophrenia is thought to result from a relative excess of central dopaminergic neuronal activity, especially in the mesolimbic-frontal cortical pathways. Dopamine antagonism by the antipsychotics causes symptoms of parkinsonism. This is probably due to nonspecific blockade of dopamine in the nigrostriatal pathways. Dopamine enhancement in treatment of parkinsonism causes some symptoms of schizophrenia. With more complete understanding of the types of dopamine receptors in specific areas of the brain and with development of drugs more specific for the various types of receptors, some of these interactive side effects may be avoided.

The term neuroleptic is used to describe the action of antipsychotic agents in suppression of spontaneous movements and complex behavior. However, spinal reflexes and unconditioned nociceptic avoidance behaviors remain intact. These drugs reduce initiative and interest in the environment and decrease displays of emotion or affect. In psychotic patients they cause a reduction in confusion and agitation with normalization of psychomotor activity. Higher intellectual functions are left intact.

The antipsychotics have no effect in treating behavioral problems of senile dementia. They have been used inappropriately for sedation in such patients.

TABLE 10–1.

Criteria for Diagnosis of Schizophrenia

At least one of the following:
Delusions
Hallucinations, especially auditory
Incoherence
Flat or inappropriate affect
Catatonia
Deterioration of previous level of functioning
Duration at least 6 months
Onset before 45 years of age
Exclusions
No preceding depressive or manic episode of extended duration
Not secondary to organic brain syndrome or mental retardation

DRUGS

The mechanism of action of the antipsychotics is thought to be an antagonism of the action of dopamine in specific areas of the central nervous system. This anti-dopaminergic action may well account for the extrapyramidal symptoms seen in persons using these drugs. Dopamine receptor antagonists are often effective as antipsychotics, and drugs that increase dopamine activity can either induce a psychosis or exacerbate a schizophrenic illness. The typical neuroleptics act on both mesolimbic and nigrostriatal dopamine pathways. The differences among drugs in this group relate to the degree of sedation and the risk of adverse effects. As with many other drugs that act in the central nervous system, receptor blockade occurs immediately, but clinical efficacy is not seen until after at least 3 weeks or more of treatment. Drugs used in treatment of the psychoses are listed in Table 10–2.

Chlorpromazine (Thorazine) was introduced in the 1950s, and since then many psychotic people have been treated effectively with this agent. This drug has had a revolutionary, and beneficial, impact on medical and psychiatric practice. Psychotic patients become less agitated and restless, and autistic patients become more responsive. These drugs differ from the sedative-hypnotics in that the patient is easily aroused, with intact intellectual functions. There is neither ataxia nor incoordination. Aggressive and impulsive behaviors are diminished and operant behavior is reduced, but spinal reflexes remain unchanged. The antipsychotics calm the patient without depression of the entire central nervous system.

Chlorpromazine is metabolized in the liver. The therapeutic effects from a single dose usually last 24 hours, allowing for once a day administration. This drug is lipid soluble and concentrates in the brain. Thus, plasma levels have little correlation with the therapeutic response. The elderly and infants have a decreased metabolic inactivation, so reduction in dosage may be required to prevent overdosing. Chlorpromazine has alpha blocking activity, which may account for the possibility of postural hypotension. Because of side effects, the elderly may respond better to lower doses

TABLE 10–2.

Antipsychotic Drugs

Drug	Total Daily Dose (mg)
Chlorpromazine (Thorazine)	200–800
Haloperidol (Haldol)	2–20
Triflupromazine (Vesprin)	20–60*
Mesoridazine besylate (Serentil)	100–400
Thioridazine (Mellaril)	200–800
Acetophenazine maleate (Tindal)	40–120
Trifluoperazine (Stelazine)	4–20
Loxapine succinate (Loxitane)	60–100
Clozapine (Clozaril)	300–600
Molindone (Moban)	15–225
Thiothixene (Navane)	6–30

*Intramuscular injection.

that are administered more frequently than once a day. Children, however, have increased metabolic inactivation.

Haloperidol (Haldol) is an antipsychotic agent that has less anticholinergic and alpha blocking activity than chlorpromazine. However, hypotension may still be a problem, as it is with chlorpromazine. Extrapyramidal symptoms are generally worse with haloperidol than with chlorpromazine. Thioridazine (Mellaril) has a lower risk of extrapyramidal side effects and less sedation than chlorpromazine or haloperidol. There are serious risks of eye damage that may limit long-term use of thioridazine.

Clozapine (Clozaril) is a new drug that may benefit those people who have not responded to chlorpromazine or haloperidol. This agent has a more selective action on the mesolimbic system. An advantage to clozapine is the low risk of development of extrapyramidal symptoms and tardive dyskinesia (see the section Adverse Effects). Most antipsychotic drugs block central dopamine receptors. Clozapine, however, is a weak dopamine receptor blocker, which may account for its causing fewer extrapyramidal symptoms than the other antipsychotics. However, there are unwanted motor effects and pronounced cardiovascular changes. The anticholinergic action of clozapine may be increased if used concurrently with other anticholinergic acting drugs. Hypotension may be exacerbated by various antihypertensives. One percent of people taking this drug may develop a blood dyscrasia, agranulocytosis, which may be fatal. However, it is most likely reversible if the drug is immediately withdrawn. Frequent monitoring of blood is required for changes in white blood cells. Currently, this drug is marketed through the Clozaril Patient Management system, which includes blood monitoring with drug distribution. The increased expense of the required monitoring and dispensing is under review.

Clozapine is rapidly absorbed from the gastrointestinal system after oral administration and is extensively metabolized by the liver. It has a half-life of 14 to 16 hours and a duration of action of greater than 24 hours. Because of its sedative side effects, it may be given at bedtime. Long-term treatment of up to 13 years has been shown to be safe and effective. Sudden discontinuation of the drug may cause withdrawal symptoms with sudden relapse in symptoms, requiring hospitalization. Except for withdrawal subsequent to aberrant blood counts, the drug should be withdrawn gradually.

Adverse effects

Side effects of the neuroleptics generally result from nonspecific receptor blockade. Blockade of cholinergic (muscarinic), noradrenergic, and dopaminergic receptors in the central and autonomic nervous systems account for most of the side effects seen with these agents. Commonly reported side effects due to anticholinergic actions are dry mouth, blurring of vision, decreased gastrointestinal activity, and sedation. Tolerance to the sedative effects usually develops within a few days.

The antipsychotics also have alpha adrenergic blocking activity, in blocking the pressor effect of norepinephrine, which may result in orthostatic hypotension and tachycardia. Strong alpha adrenergic blocking activity is seen with triflupromazine and chlorpromazine; weak activity, with trifluoperazine and clozapine. Tolerance to these effects also may develop with continued use. However, postural hypotension may persist in the elderly, with its attendant risk of falls and fractures.

The antidopamine actions are more serious. Acute dystonia, akathisia, and parkinsonism appear early with antipsychotic treatment. The acute dystonia may appear transiently, and disappear without additional treatment. Akathisia or motor restlessness usually responds to a reduction in the antipsychotic dose; however, dose reduction may compromise treatment of the psychosis. The extrapyramidal symptoms are indistinguishable from those of parkinsonism and may be the most bothersome of the side effects. The symptoms may respond to benztropine mesylate (Cogentin) or trihexyphenidyl (Artane).

The antipsychotics also may cause tardive dyskinesia, especially in the elderly, which may not be reversible. This may develop during treatment with an antipsychotic or after treatment is discontinued. Patients over 60 years old, especially those with preexisting central nervous system disease, are at greater risk to develop tardive dyskinesia. This is a choreiform disorder, with oral-facial dyskinesia, choreoathetosis, lip smacking and sucking, lateral jaw movements, and tongue darting. To reduce the risk of tardive dyskinesia, the lowest possible effective dose should be used. Drug holidays from the antipsychotic do not appear to prevent the development of tardive dyskinesia. There is no effective drug treatment for tardive dyskinesia.

Some antipsychotics lower the seizure threshold. In a patient susceptible to seizures, for example those with epilepsy, selection of the appropriate neuroleptic agent should be made with regard to the effect on the seizure threshold. Thioridazine has a minimal effect on this threshold, whereas chlorpromazine may predispose epileptics to seizures.

It is not possible to predict an individual's response to any antipsychotic drug. Different people respond differently. Selection of a particular drug may be based on the potential of certain side effects and the experience of the prescribing physician.

The antipsychotics have a high therapeutic index. Overdose is rarely fatal, unless administered in combination with alcohol or other central nervous system sedatives.

PHYSICAL THERAPY NOTES

Physical therapy treatment of patients with uncontrolled psychoses is very difficult. The patient's lack of attention and frequent belligerence can cause great difficulty in maintaining any type of patient interactive program.

As with any drug that has the potential to cause hypotension, specific attention should be given to prevention of injury to the patient from falls. Assistance in ambulation may be appropriate, especially after the initial administration of the antipsychotic drug.

Because development of extrapyramidal symptoms is a common side effect of most of the antipsychotics, the physical therapist should be attentive to the appearance of these motor symptoms. Akinesia, muscle rigidity, tremors, and other motor symptoms are the most likely to occur. These symptoms generally occur within a month after initiation of drug treatment.

Psychoses may develop from chronic administration of glucocorticoids, as may be used in treatment of chronic inflammatory diseases. This is more likely with oral administration every day than with alternate-day therapy or with topical application.

LEARNING OBJECTIVES

1. Understand the uses of antipsychotics in treatment of psychoses.
2. Explain the transient and persistent side effects of the antipsychotics.
3. List the side effects of the antipsychotics resulting from antidopamine activity.
4. List the side effects of the antipsychotics resulting from anticholinergic actions.
5. List the side effects of the antipsychotics resulting from alpha adrenergic blocking activity.

ADDITIONAL READINGS

1. Baldessarini RJ, Tarsy D: Relationship of the actions of neuroleptic drugs to the pathophysiology of tardive dyskinesia. *Int Rev Neurobiol* 1979; 21:1–45.
2. Coyle JT: The clinical use of antipsychotic medications. *Med Clin North Am* 1982; 66:993–1009.
3. Johnson DAW: Pharmacological treatment of patients with schizophrenia. *Drugs* 1990; 39:481–488.

Disorders of Movement

Chapter 11

Drugs Used in Treatment of Parkinson's Disease

Over a half million people, mostly age 55 and older, are affected with Parkinson's disease. Parkinson's disease is most likely due to a lack of dopamine action in the basal ganglia. This is probably the result of a degeneration of the dopaminergic nigrostriatal tract. The cause is not known; however, it does not appear to have a genetic basis. Recent research regarding the mechanism of induction of a parkinson-like syndrome by 1-methyl-4-phenyl-1,2,3,6-tetrahydropyridine (MPTP) has led to the speculation that the cause of Parkinson's disease is a free radical toxin, either endogenous or exogenous. Parkinson's disease is characterized by the tetrad of bradykinesia, rigidity, tremors at rest, and postural defects. There is also increased sweating and increased salivation, possibly due to an increased acetylcholine activity. There are psychiatric disturbances associated with Parkinson's disease. Depression is frequently seen, and it may be part of the disease process itself, rather than a reaction to the disabling aspects of the disease. Depression in patients with Parkinson's disease is worse than is seen in other disabling diseases, such as arthritis. Alterations in sensation, such as numbness, aching, or burning, have also been reported. Whether this is the result of a change in the sensory system or the integration systems is not known.

The hallmarks of Parkinson's disease are bradykinesia, rigidity, tremors at rest, and postural deficits.

1. Bradykinesia is not only slowness of movement but also a paucity and imprecision of movement. There is a loss of associated movements—such as arm swinging during gait, or gesticulations, eye blinks, and facial movements during speech. This latter causes the masked facies. Repetitive movements are slowed and irregular. Fine motor coordination diminishes. Movements requiring great organizations, such as getting up from a chair and getting into or out of a car, become difficult. Whether the deficit is in planning or execution is not known.

TABLE 11–1.

Anticholinergic Drugs

Drug	Total Daily Dose (mg)	Times/Day
Trihexyphenidyl (Artane)	12–15	3
Benztropine mesylate (Cogentin)	1–2	1
Ethopropazine (Parsidol)	50–600	2
Orphenadrine (Norflex)	200	2
Biperiden (Akineton)	8–16	3–4

2. Rigidity is the result of increased muscle tone, with co-contraction of both the flexors and the extensors. There is a cogwheel or ratchet resistance to passive movement. This rigidity is not velocity dependent, as is seen in spasticity.

3. Tremors at rest are very common in Parkinson's disease, and may be one of the early signs. These diminish with voluntary movements, and with sleep, but worsen with emotional stress. This is seen as a "pill-rolling" movement of the hands. The abnormal movements may range from a source of embarrassment to a major physical disability. The head is rarely involved. Head tremors are apparent in essential tremor and they worsen with sustained effort. Essential tremor vanishes with sleep, also.

4. The postural defects appear later in the course of the disease. The person demonstrates a progressively stooped posture and a festinating gait. The postural instability that occurs can be very disabling. Walking aids are generally not much use because they are difficult for the person to handle and they do not prevent backward falls. The person has difficulty in initiating gait, difficulty in turning, and difficulty in stopping.

PHARMACOLOGIC MANAGEMENT OF PARKINSON'S DISEASE

The output from the basal ganglia appears to be due to the balance between the inhibitory dopaminergic and the excitatory cholinergic pathways. Drugs used to treat Parkinson's disease can attempt either to increase the level of dopamine in the striatum or to decrease the amount of acetylcholine activity. Either approach is an attempt to restore the appropriate dopamine:acetylcholine ratio.

Anticholinergic Drugs

An anticholinergic drug may be the drug of choice early in the disease (Table 11–1). Trihexyphenidyl (Artane) is used in treating the early stage of Parkinson's disease in an attempt to reduce the effects of acetylcholine. This treatment does not affect the dopamine levels. By reducing the effect of acetylcholine, the anticholinergic drug allows for more apparent dopamine activity, even from the reduced dopamine that is still present. Anticholinergic drugs are more effective in reducing tremors than

TABLE 11–2.

Dopaminergic Drugs

Drug	Total Daily Dose	Times/Day
Levodopa (Larodopa)	8 g	Several
Sinemet*	300–800 mg†	3
Bromocriptine (Parlodel)	100 mg	2
Amantadine (Symmetrel)	200 mg	2
Selegiline (Eldepryl)	10 mg	1–2

*Carbidopa and levodopa in combination.
†Levodopa.

altering the rigidity and bradykinesia. Trihexyphenidyl also may be used to treat drug-induced extrapyramidal symptoms associated with long-term treatment with antipsychotics.

Adverse effects from anticholinergic treatment are as expected: dry mouth, urinary retention, and constipation. Confusion, delirium, and hallucinations also may be seen. These side effects are generally not as disturbing to the patient as the disease itself, and may disappear with continuing treatment. With progression of the disease, and further reduction in the endogenous dopamine, the anticholinergic drugs generally lose their effectiveness.

Dopaminergic Drugs

Dopaminergic drugs are those that exert their actions through the dopamine receptor (Table 11–2). Dopamine, itself, cannot be used as a drug because it does not cross the blood-brain barrier. Levodopa (Larodopa) is a precursor to dopamine that does cross the blood-brain barrier. Levodopa is converted to dopamine by L-amino acid decarboxylase, both in the peripheral tissues and in the brain neurons. The peripheral production of dopamine does nothing for the treatment of Parkinson's disease, and may account for metabolism of over 90% of an administered dose. This peripheral metabolism is responsible for high doses of levodopa required to get sufficient amounts of levodopa into the brain. The short elimination half-life (1 to 1½ hours) of levodopa also is due to its peripheral metabolism.

The combination of carbidopa, a peripheral decarboxylase inhibitor, with levodopa, allows for lower doses of levodopa, and decreases the side effects related to peripheral actions of dopamine. This combination is called Sinemet. Carbidopa, itself, has no known pharmacologic effects and does not cross the blood-brain barrier. Conversion of levodopa in the basal ganglia is not inhibited by carbidopa. Sinemet may be used in combination with any other drug used to treat Parkinson's disease except levodopa, and the dosage is reduced as necessary.

Adverse effects resulting from levodopa use include nausea, vomiting, and anorexia, and occur in 80% of patients. Tolerance to these adverse effects may develop. Giving the drug with food may reduce the incidence of these effects; however, administration with meals may also reduce the amount of the absorbed dose. Transient tachycardia may occur because of dopamine stimulation of beta-1 receptors in the heart. A beta blocker may be used if treatment of this seems necessary. Orthostatic hypotension develops in 30% of patients taking levodopa. Continued use may result in tolerance to this. Excess daytime sleepiness may occur, and, again, may decrease with continued treatment.

Half the patients taking levodopa develop abnormal involuntary movements (dyskinesias) after about 3 months of treatment. These are variable in type, and may be evident as faciolingual tics, grimacing, head bobbing, and rocking movements of the trunk or extremities. Tolerance does not develop. Reduction of the dose may reduce their appearance, but this also reduces therapeutic efficacy. Psychiatric disturbances such as hallucinations, paranoia, mania, and depression may develop in patients on levodopa therapy, and again, reduction in dose or complete withdrawal may be warranted. Usually, people respond to levodopa for only about 3 years. The 3-year period seems to relate to the duration of levodopa administration, rather than to the duration of the disease. The conversion of levodopa to dopamine in the striatum requires viable neurons. For this reason, many physicians will prescribe an anticholinergic early in the disease and for as long as it works, until levodopa is finally prescribed.

An "on-off" phenomenon is frequently seen in patients taking levodopa, with oscillations in severity of symptoms, from full function and mobility to almost complete immobility. This may occur within short time periods, even during a single day. This phenomenon seems to be related to the blood levels of levodopa. Intervals between drug administrations may need to be shortened. The "on-off" phenomenon also may relate to interference with gastrointestinal absorption. The pharmacologic effects of levodopa are not seen in healthy persons or in non-basal ganglia-related neurologic diseases.

Other drugs may be used that act through the dopaminergic pathway. Bromocriptine (Parlodel) is a dopamine agonist and has shown some success in treatment of Parkinson's disease. Amantadine (Symmetrel) is an antiviral agent that releases dopamine from nerve terminals and delays reuptake. This drug may be used in combination with levodopa, and the combination may allow for a reduction in levodopa dose and consequent reduction in side effects. Amantadine is relatively free of side effects but loses efficacy in 6 to 8 weeks. Episodic use may restore efficacy. Adverse effects from long-term use of amantadine include livedo reticularis, a purplish mottling of the skin, in response to local release of norepinephrine. This is reversible when the drug is stopped. Also, dry mouth and constipation may be seen. Amantadine also may be used to treat drug-induced extrapyramidal symptoms.

A very recently released drug, selegiline (Eldepryl), has shown great potential in treatment of Parkinson's disease. Selegiline was formerly called deprenyl. This is an inhibitor of monoamine oxidase-B, an enzyme responsible for degrading dopamine in the central nervous system. Preliminary clinical trials suggest that this drug may slow progression of the disease. With a limited number of patients tested, there have been no serious side effects. Side effects of other monoamine oxidase inhibitors used in treatment of the psychoses are not seen.

PHYSICAL THERAPY NOTES

Because of the nature of the motor disturbances in Parkinson's disease and their interference with normal function, physical therapists are frequently called upon to treat these patients. The goal of physical therapy treatment is to maintain as much function as possible over the longest time. Physical therapy treatment does not alter the course of the disease, but may extend the functional time for the patient. With continuing development of new pharmacologic treatments, maintenance of function over longer times is possible.

Physical therapy treatment is aimed at decreasing the movement dysfunctions that interfere with normal function. If the patient's functional ability has degenerated prior to beginning physical therapy, then restoration is necessary. Obviously, it is easier to maintain current abilities than to restore lost function. Exercise is important to maintain flexibility and to prevent the sequelae of deconditioning.

Postural instability may present a challenge to the therapist. Stimulation of balance reactions when protective reactions are lost requires an innovative treatment plan. Dizziness and postural hypotension as side effects from some drugs used to treat this disease pose a danger to the patient. In those patients having serious problems with postural stability, exercises that require minimum balance, for example, done in a wheelchair, might be recommended.

The "on-off" phenomenon with wide swings in motor function can interfere with treatment planning. The patient may vary in functional mobility even within short time periods. Flexibility in treatment planning and scheduling is required for optimal benefits to the patient.

Bradykinesia and rigidity both contribute to the inability to initiate movements. Correct positioning of the body before a movement is initiated may allow the person to compensate for some of this loss. Patients may have lost some of the "feel" for the correct posture. Incorrect posture in sitting may prevent a patient from rising to the standing position.

The flexed and fixed posture inhibits natural movement. Treatment programs to increase rotation and to increase reciprocal rhythmical movements in walking may facilitate more normal postures. The flexed posture, with rigidity, may compromise respiratory function. Extension exercises should be emphasized.

Tremors at rest, although they do not directly interfere with function, may make the person hesitant about appearing in public. These tremors are increased by stress and anxiety.

LEARNING OBJECTIVES

1. Describe the neurochemical changes in the brain that correlate with Parkinson's disease.
2. List the classes of drugs used to treat Parkinson's disease and the rationale behind the use of each class of drugs.

3. Understand the progressive nature of Parkinson's disease. Discuss the disease symptoms vs. drug side effects.
4. Discuss the side effects of the drugs used to treat Parkinson's disease and how these may affect total treatment of the patient.

ADDITIONAL READINGS

1. Coleman RJ: Rational management of the "on-off" syndrome in Parkinson's disease. *Q J Med* 1990; 74:121–131.
2. Halliwell B: Oxidants and the central nervous system: Some fundamental questions. *Acta Neurol Scand* 1989; 126:23–33.
3. Heinonen EH, Rinne UK: Selegiline in the treatment of Parkinson's disease. *Acta Neurol Scand* 1989; 126:103–111.
4. Nutt JG: Parkinson's disease: Evaluation and therapeutic strategy. *Hosp Pract* 1987; 22(Apr):107–136.
5. The Parkinson Study Group: Effect of deprenyl on the progression of disability in early Parkinson's disease. *N Engl J Med* 1989; 321:1364–1371.
6. Shoulson I, and the Parkinson Study Group: Deprenyl and tocopherol antioxidative therapy of parkinsonism (DATATOP). *Acta Neurol Scand* 1989; 126:171–175.
7. Steg G, Ingvarsson PE, Johnels B, et al: Objective measurement of motor disability in Parkinson's disease. *Acta Neurol Scand* 1989; 126:67–75.

Chapter 12

Antiepileptic Drugs

Seizures refer to electroclinical events, whereas epilepsy indicates a tendency for recurrent seizures. Not all seizures are due to epilepsy. Epilepsies are a group of chronic central nervous system disorders having in common the occurrence of sudden and transitory episodes of abnormal phenomena of motor, sensory, autonomic, or psychic origin. These are nearly always associated with abnormal and excessive electrical activity of brain cells, especially in the cerebral cortex. Epilepsy can be associated with loss of consciousness and possibly uncontrolled muscular activity, twitching, or convulsions. The types of epilepsies are identified from the electroencephalographic pattern and from clinical manifestations. Accurate diagnosis is important because pharmacologic therapy is selective. Although the causative factor in epilepsy is not always evident, it may occur subsequent to fever, head trauma, or viral infections.

TYPES OF EPILEPSIES

Tonic-clonic epilepsy, or grand mal, is usually a sequence of maximal tonic spasms of all body musculature, followed by synchronous clonic jerking and a prolonged depression of all central functions, resulting in loss of consciousness. Status epilepticus is a series of grand mal convulsions and constitutes a medical emergency.

Absence seizures or petit mal are characterized by an abrupt and brief loss of consciousness and memory, with usually some symmetrical clonic motor activity, from eye blinking to jerking of the body, or there may be no motor activity. These are not convulsions. Absence seizures begin in childhood or early adolescence. They have a disruptive effect on normal activities, so they should be treated. There is the possibility of accidental injury during the loss of awareness. A child with absence seizures is at a particular risk for injury during unprotected activities, such as crossing a street, riding a bike, or climbing a tree.

Simple partial epilepsies have various manifestations, without impairment of consciousness, including convulsions confined to a single limb or muscle group.

TABLE 12–1.

Antiepileptic Drugs

Drug	Total Daily Dose*	Times/Day
Phenobarbital (Luminal)	3–6 mg/kg†	2
	60–250 mg‡	1
Phenytoin (Dilantin)	4–8 mg/kg†	2–3
	300–400 mg‡	1–3
Carbamazepine (Tegretol)	400–800 mg†	3–4
	800–1,200‡	
Ethosuximide (Zarontin)	20 mg/kg†	1
	250–1,000 mg‡	
Valproic acid (Depakene)	1,000–3,000 mg‡	1–3
Clonazepam (Klonopin)	.01–.02 mg/kg†	3
	<20 mg‡	2–3

*For discussion, see text.
†Children.
‡Adults.

Psychomotor epilepsies are attacks of confused behavior, generally with impairment of consciousness. The person is usually amnesic about these.

PHARMACOLOGIC MANAGEMENT OF EPILEPSIES

The term antiepileptic is used here to denote a drug used in treatment of epileptic disorders. It does not imply an effect against the underlying disease process. Antiepileptic agents may have effects on the neurons of the seizure foci to prevent their excessive discharge or they may reduce the spread of excitation from the seizure foci. Most agents currently in use appear to work through the latter mechanism, that is, to reduce the spread of the abnormal electrical activity. The ideal drug would suppress all seizures without unwanted adverse effects. In reality, the individual drugs may fail to control all seizures and they can cause adverse effects, from minimal impairment of the central nervous system to death from aplastic anemia or hepatic failure. The mechanism of action of any of the drugs in chronic therapy in a particular type of epilepsy is unknown. All the drugs have a greater frequency of side effects on initiation of therapy. For this reason, drug therapy is generally initiated at lower than maintenance levels, and the dose is gradually increased until seizures are under control, the maximum recommended dose is reached, or side effects occur. Drugs used in management of epilepsies are listed in Table 12–1. The doses listed are those required for maintenance therapy. Initiation doses are generally lower.

Phenobarbital

The first effective antiepileptic was phenobarbital (Luminal). It is an anticonvulsant at lower doses than are used for sedative-hypnotic purposes. However, sedation may limit its use in some sensitive people. Tolerance to the sedative effect may develop with continued use. Phenobarbital is effective for generalized tonic-clonic and partial seizures, and may be used in combination with other drugs. It is ineffective against absence seizures but may be used to prevent emergence of tonic-clonic epilepsy. It also may be used in psychomotor epilepsy. Its mechanism of action is thought to be due to membrane stabilization. Its use in children is controversial. It may cause irritability and hyperreactivity, other mood and behavioral problems, and cognitive dysfunction. There have also been reports of decreased mental development in children who have been treated chronically with phenobarbital. In the elderly it may cause agitation, insomnia, and confusion. Long-term treatment with phenobarbital may cause connective tissue changes, causing Dupuytren's contracture, frozen shoulder, and generalized aches and pains.

Phenobarbital is absorbed from the small intestine, and the peak serum concentration is reached in about 4 hours. The half-life varies from 24 to 140 hours. The drug is about 50% bound to protein, so the free drug concentration may increase in diseases that produce a low plasma protein concentration. It is metabolized in the liver and excreted by the kidneys. This drug also induces the liver microsomal enzyme system. This may shorten the half-life of phenobarbital, as well as that of other drugs metabolized by this liver enzyme system.

Although systemic side effects are rare during treatment with phenobarbital, annoying neurologic and psychologic toxicity is frequent. At normal doses, adverse changes in affect, behavior, and cognitive function are often encountered. At high doses, nystagmus, dysarthria, incoordination, and ataxia may be seen. The hallmark of phenobarbital toxicity is sedation. This may occur at the onset of treatment, but tolerance generally develops, even as the dose is increased. Abrupt discontinuance of phenobarbital may cause withdrawal symptoms such as anxiety, emotional lability, insomnia, tremors, diaphoresis, confusion, and possibly, seizures. Tapering the dose may alleviate these withdrawal systems.

Phenytoin

Phenytoin (Dilantin) is also a primary drug in the treatment of tonic-clonic and psychomotor seizures. This drug does not have the potential for sedation as does phenobarbital. It decreases hyperexcitability of nerve cells by making them more hyperpolarized. The cells have a longer refractory period to subsequent stimulation. Phenytoin reduces the spread of the seizure process from an active, abnormally firing epileptic focus into adjacent normal brain tissue. This drug has a high therapeutic index.

Phenytoin is absorbed from the intestine and about 90% is bound to plasma protein, at the same site as valproic acid (Depakene). The plasma half-life after oral administration is about 22 hours, with a wide variation seen among patients.

Adverse effects from chronic administration of phenytoin at low levels of toxicity include visual disturbances such as nystagmus and diplopia, and cerebellar-vestibular effects such as dizziness, ataxia, vertigo, and postural imbalance. Higher levels of toxicity are evident as dysarthria, incoordination, and significant unsteadiness. Drowsiness, lethargy, and coma are seen at very toxic levels. Gingival hyperplasia caused by phenytoin may be controlled with meticulous oral hygiene. This is more common and severe in younger patients, under 21 years of age, and is less frequently seen in adults. Drug allergy and skin rashes may develop, which necessitate withdrawal of the drug. Mild hirsutism is common. Phenytoin can produce irritability, hallucinations, and even psychotic reactions. Megaloblastic anemia is seen only rarely. Because of the different mechanisms of action of phenobarbital and phenytoin, they may be administered concurrently. The advantage of using lower doses of each agent, compared to single agent treatment, is to reduce the incidence and severity of side effects.

Carbamazepine

Carbamazepine (Tegretol) is used for generalized tonic-clonic seizures and for simple and complex partial seizures. Treatment of the latter is generally less effective than treatment of the other epilepsies. However, carbamazepine is more effective than phenobarbital against partial seizures. Carbamazepine has fewer side effects than phenobarbital in children. Carbamazepine also is used for trigeminal neuralgia.

Carbomazepine is metabolized by liver enzymes, with a half-life of 36 hours. This can be decreased to 24 hours after induction of the liver metabolizing enzymes, that is, concurrent use with phenobarbital.

Chronic administration of carbamazepine is associated with drowsiness, vertigo, ataxia, and diplopia. However, cognitive, affective, and behavioral effects are uncommon. There is less psychologic and behavioral toxicity than with phenytoin and phenobarbital. In fact, there may be improved mood and activity levels, with improved alertness and mental functioning. There may be a reduction in apathy and lack of initiative, a quickening of thought and action, and an improvement in attendant concentration. The slow-release form may cause less daily fluctuations in serum levels. Although there are a multiplicity of side effects, the serious ones are rare. Compared with other drug treatments, carbamazepine is considered relatively safe. Neurologic side effects are the most common, with nausea, headache, dizziness, and diplopia most frequently reported. Tolerance usually develops rapidly, allowing continuance of the drug. The elderly are more sensitive to neurologic side effects. Rashes may be seen, but are transient. There is also a possibility of hematologic toxicity associated with this agent, but it seems to be rare.

Ethosuximide

Ethosuximide (Zarontin) is the drug of choice in treating absence seizures, without tonic-clonic seizures. More than 50% of these patients can be controlled by this agent. Although phenytoin and phenobarbital are ineffective in absence seizures, they may be used in combination with ethosuximide in order to guard against appearance of general tonic-clonic seizures.

Ethosuximide is minimally (<10%) bound to proteins. It is slowly cleared from the plasma, with a half-life of greater than 50 hours in adults, and of about 30 hours in children.

Chronic treatment with ethosuximide has been associated with gastrointestinal symptoms such as anorexia, nausea, and vomiting. These are mostly dose related and may be alleviated by dose reduction. A persistent headache also may be seen with ethosuximide use. Central nervous system symptoms of drowsiness and lethargy may occur. A parkinson-like syndrome has been reported to develop with long-term use of ethosuximide.

Valproic Acid

Valproic acid (Depakene) can be used in treatment of absence, general tonic-clonic, and myoclonic seizures. Although the adverse effects of ethosuximide are generally fewer or less serious than those of valproic acid, these two drugs can be used in combination. Valproic acid and ethosuximide are equally effective in absence seizures. Valproic acid is the drug of choice in myoclonic seizures, occurring with degenerative central nervous system disease or postanoxic encephalopathy. However, these disorders may be refractory to treatment. Valproic acid is used in patients with tonic-clonic seizures, appearing alone or with absence and/or myoclonic seizures. The effect of therapy may not be apparent for several weeks after initiating treatment.

Valproic acid is rapidly absorbed from the intestinal tract, with a peak plasma concentration seen about 2 hours after oral administration. The enteric coated preparations, utilized to reduce gastrointestinal discomfort, have variable absorption, with peak concentrations seen from 3 to 8 hours after administration. Valproic acid is extensively protein-bound (about 90%), and is metabolized by the liver. The half-life is from 12 to 16 hours.

Gastrointestinal disturbances are most commonly noted with initiation of valproic acid treatment, and can be circumvented by giving the drug after meals, or using an enteric coated preparation. Side effects of valproic acid are tremors and alopecia. There may be a dose related tremor of an essential type, but it is rarely sufficiently severe to limit treatment. Valproic acid can cause an increased appetite and subsequent weight gain, if conscious control of diet is not obtained. As with carbamazepine, cognitive, affective, and behavioral effects are uncommon. Idiosyncrasies seen are neutropenia and bone marrow suppression. Thrombocytopenia also may be seen. A serious toxicity of valproic acid is liver failure. This generally is manifested during the first few months of treatment. Liver function tests should be administered prior to therapy to form a baseline, and then at regular intervals after therapy has been initiated.

Clonazepam

Clonazepam (Klonopin) is a benzodiazepine that is effective in treatment of absence seizures. Tolerance does develop to its antiepileptic activity within about 3 to 6 months, so its use in chronic treatment is limited. The side effects are characteristic of the benzodiazepines, such as drowsiness, ataxia, and changes in mood. The central nervous system depressive effects are potentiated by other central nervous depressants, such as alcohol, barbiturates, and the antidepressants. Behavioral disturbances are more common in children and may be seen as hyperactivity and increased aggressiveness. Severe toxicity is rare.

PHYSICAL THERAPY NOTES

The use of antiepileptic drugs to prevent seizures following head trauma is fairly common; however, few well-designed clinical studies have been tested. The sedative side effects may interfere with physical therapy treatment.

Children with absence seizures that are not completely under control may exhibit what appear to be attention lapses. These can be dangerous in an unprotected situation, such as when crossing a street.

LEARNING OBJECTIVES

1. Understand the various types of epilepsy.
2. Know the classes of drug used to treat these disorders, and their side effects.

ADDITIONAL READINGS

1. Bleck TP: Convulsive disorders: The use of anticonvulsant drugs. *Clin Neuropharmacol* 1990; 13:198–209.
2. Bleck TP, Klawans HL: Convulsive disorders: Mechanisms of epilepsy and anticonvulsant action. *Clin Neuropharmacol* 1990; 13:121–128.
3. Dichter MA, Ayala GF: Cellular mechanisms of epilepsy: A status report. *Science* 1987; 237:157–164.
4. Farwell JR, Lee YJ, Hirtz DG, et al: Phenobarbital for febrile seizures—effects on intelligence and on seizure recurrence. *N Engl J Med* 1990; 322:364–369.
5. Scheuer ML, Pedley TA: The evaluation and treatment of seizures. *N Engl J Med* 1990; 323:1468–1474.
6. Temkin NR, Dikmen SS, Wilensky AJ, et al: A randomized, double-blind study of phenytoin for the prevention of post-traumatic seizures. *N Engl J Med* 1990; 323:497–502.

Chapter 13 _____

Spasticity and Skeletal Muscle Relaxants

Skeletal muscle relaxants are used in an attempt to treat spasticity. Currently, there is no completely satisfactory form of therapy for alleviation of skeletal muscle spasticity that does not cause muscular weakness in nonspastic muscles. All skeletal muscles, including muscles of respiration, can be affected by the treatment. The order of muscular weakness affected by treatment is first extraocular, then hands and feet, head and neck, abdominal and extremities, and diaphragm. Spasticity is a poorly understood dysfunction of descending pathways, especially the corticospinal, reticulospinal, and vestibulospinal pathways. The peripheral reflex arcs, although hyperactive because of abnormal control from higher centers, are not primarily involved. Nevertheless, sites in these arcs, skin afferents, spindle afferents, interneurons, and efferents to intrafusal and extrafusal fibers, may be pharmacologic targets.

DRUG TREATMENT OF SPASTICITY

Dantrolene (Dantrium) is a direct acting skeletal muscle relaxant, in that it blocks calcium release from the sarcoplasmic reticulum. In patients with upper motor neuron lesions, dantrolene decreases spasticity, which increases functional capacity. It is used in treatment of spastic diseases, such as multiple sclerosis and athetoid cerebral palsy. Tolerance to its actions does not develop. Adverse effects include a dose dependent skeletal muscular weakness of nonspastic muscles and liver dysfunction. The generalized muscle weakness may prove as much of a detriment to function as the spasticity. Dantrolene is especially useful in nonambulatory patients when spasticity hinders nursing care. It produces comparable relaxation with less sedation than does diazepam (Valium).

Diazepam (Valium) is a centrally acting skeletal muscle relaxant. It acts in the spinal cord and enhances the efficiency of gamma aminobutyric acid (GABA) transmission. Thus, it enhances presynaptic inhibition of afferent neuronal terminals. It is used principally in treatment of muscle spasm resulting from trauma, tension, or overexertion. It is used to control flexor and extensor spasms. Spasticity and athetosis in cerebral palsy also may be treated with diazepam. Effectiveness of therapy for longer than 4 months has not been assessed. The most troublesome adverse effect is drowsiness, which is dose dependent. Because of its central nervous system depressant action, it should not be used with other central nervous system depressants. Tolerance develops to both therapeutic and side effects. Other benzodiazepines have skeletal muscle relaxant activity and all have the same indications and contraindications.

Another centrally acting agent is baclofen (Lioresal), which is a derivative of GABA. It exerts its antispastic effects by decreasing release of excitatory neurotransmitters from primary afferent terminals and thus depressing monosynaptic and polysynaptic transmission in the spinal cord. It reduces EPSPs in motor neurons in the ventral horn without affecting membrane potential. Because it is effective in patients with complete spinal transections, the primary site of action seems to be the spinal cord. It is useful for treating spasticity in multiple sclerosis and spinal cord injury. It is not appropriate for cerebral palsy or stroke. It reduces the frequency and the severity of flexor or extensor spasms and reduces increased flexor tone. Adverse effects are drowsiness and muscular weakness, which may limit its usefulness in ambulatory patients. The threshold for initiation of seizures may be lowered in patients with epilepsy. Sudden withdrawal after chronic administration may cause auditory and visual hallucinations, anxiety, and tachycardia.

DRUG TREATMENT OF ACUTE MUSCLE SPASMS

Drugs for acute muscle spasms are chlorzoxazone (Parafon Forte, Paraflex), cyclobenzaprine (Flexeril), and carisoprodol (Soma). These probably act at the central nervous system. They appear to block interneuronal activity in the spinal cord. They do not act at the neuromuscular junction or directly on skeletal muscle. Their efficacy in treatment of acute muscle spasms is not established. The sedative side effects promote rest, which itself may be effective in treatment of acute muscle spasms. Rest and heat relieve discomfort. Acute muscle spasms resulting from trauma heal spontaneously, provided there is no further injury.

PHYSICAL THERAPY NOTES

The use of skeletal muscle relaxants for treating spasticity are a mixed blessing for physical therapists. On the one hand, spasticity is reduced; however, there can be unwanted side effects. Dantrolene, which is a direct acting relaxant, also reduces tone in nonspastic muscles. This can possibly reduce overall function of the patient. However, if the patient is nonambulatory, the reduction in spasticity will allow for more effective treatment, maintenance of range of motion, and so forth.

Diazepam, a centrally acting skeletal muscle relaxant, has the side effect of drowsiness, which obviously may interfere with physical therapy treatment. The effectiveness of long-term treatment, that is, longer than 4 months, has not been evaluated. Tolerance does develop to therapeutic effects. The centrally acting agents may be useful in treating acute muscle spasms resulting from direct trauma or overexertion.

LEARNING OBJECTIVES

1. Understand the differences between direct acting and centrally acting relaxants.
2. Know the reasons for prescribing skeletal muscle relaxants.
3. Describe the effects from long-term use of drugs used in treatment of spasticity and acute muscle spasm.
4. Explain the benefits and drawbacks of pharmacologic treatment of spasticity, from a clinician's point of view.

ADDITIONAL READINGS

1. Pinder RM, Brogden RN, Speight TM, et al: Dantrolene sodium: A review of its pharmacological properties and therapeutic efficacy in spasticity. *Drugs* 1977; 13:3–23.
2. Wroblewski B, Glenn MB: Antispasticity medication in the patient with traumatic brain injury. *J Head Trauma Rehabil* 1986; 1:71–72.
3. Young RR, Delwaide PJ: Spasticity. *N Engl J Med* 1981; 304:28–33, 96–99.

PART V

Inflammatory/Immune Diseases

Chapter 14 _____

Non-Narcotic Analgesics and Nonsteroidal Anti-Inflammatory Drugs

Non-narcotic analgesics are used for relief of mild to moderate pain. Pain derived from inflammation or tissue injury, mainly related to the musculoskeletal system, is particularly amenable to treatment with these drugs. On the other hand, the non-narcotics are not effective against deep, visceral pain originating from the hollow organs. In this group of non-narcotic drugs are included the nonaspirin drug acetaminophen, and aspirin and the aspirin-like compounds. The advantage of these non-narcotic agents is that chronic use does not lead to tolerance or addiction. Most of these agents are also antipyretic, in that they will lower an elevated body temperature. However, they have no direct effect on normal body temperature at usual doses.

Inflammation is caused by release of chemicals from tissues and from migrating white blood cells in response to cellular injury. The injury may be of any nature, such as from bacteria, trauma, heat, or chemicals. The four signs of inflammation are redness, heat, pain, and swelling. Injury to any cells, except erythrocytes, activates the enzyme phospholipase in the cell membrane, which causes the release of arachidonic acid from the membrane phospholipids. Arachidonic acid can be metabolized by two enzymatic pathways (Fig 14–1). The lipoxygenase pathway synthesizes the leukotrienes, which are involved in many pathologic responses. The various leukotrienes can interact with platelets, modulate vascular tone, increase vascular permeability, and affect other aspects of inflammation. The leukotrienes, however, do not produce fever. The second pathway, mediated by the cyclooxygenase enzyme, also called prostaglandin synthetase, synthesizes the formation of the various prostaglandins and thromboxane and prostacyclin. Figure 14–1 depicts the pathways of arachidonic acid metabolism that are amenable to pharmacologic inhibition.

Aspirin and aspirin-like drugs are referred to as the nonsteroidal anti-inflammatory drugs (NSAIDs) to differentiate these agents from the glucocorticoids, the steroidal anti-

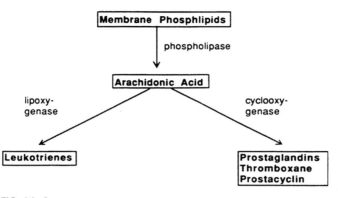

FIG 14–1.
Enzymatic pathways of arachidonic acid metabolism.
Phospholipase releases arachidonic acid from the membrane. The
cyclooxygenase and the lipoxygenase enzymes stimulate the
synthesis of prostanoids and leukotrienes, respectively, from
arachidonic acid. Aspirin and the other NSAIDs inhibit the
cyclooxygenase enzyme.

inflammatory drugs. These latter will be discussed in Chapter 15. The currently available nonsteroidal anti-inflammatory agents inhibit the cyclooxygenase enzyme, but have no apparent effect on the lipoxygenase enzyme. Other chemicals released during the inflammatory response include histamine, the kinins, interleukin 1, and factors that stimulate the bone marrow to produce more circulating neutrophils and monocytes. Interleukin 1 is also called endogenous pyrogen and is thought to be responsible for producing fever. There is a redundancy in the actions of these various chemicals, in that inhibiting only one does very little to inhibit the total process.

Aspirin and the other NSAIDs irreversibly inhibit the cyclooxygenase enzyme in platelet membranes, thus inhibiting platelet reactivity. Due to this antiplatelet effect, they are used after myocardial infarction, transient ischemic attacks, or other situations where inhibition of platelet activity is desired.

ACETAMINOPHEN

Acetaminophen (Tylenol, Datril, Excedrin, and others) has been on the market for decades; however, its mechanism of action is not known. It is effective against mild to moderate pain and is effective in reducing fever. Its antipyretic and analgesic activities are about the same as those of aspirin; however, it is not anti-inflammatory and does not reduce platelet activity. There is no gastrointestinal irritation associated with acetaminophen; however, chronic overuse has been associated with renal toxicity. Serious hepatic toxicity is associated with acute overdose. For adults a single dose of 500 to 1,000 mg is usually effective, with a recommended total daily dose not to exceed 4,000 mg. For children a single dose of 40 to 480 mg, depending on age and weight, with no more than 5 doses within 24 hours, is recommended. Acetaminophen is an effective substitute for aspirin for antipyresis and analgesia, especially for those people for whom aspirin is contraindicated. Aspirin is contraindicated in those with gastric irritation from aspirin; if the bleeding time is prolonged and platelet inhibition inappropriate; and in children, and possibly teenagers, with flulike symptoms and the possibility of Reye's syndrome.

NONSTEROIDAL ANTI-INFLAMMATORY DRUGS

Aspirin and other NSAIDs reduce fever (antipyretic), reduce pain (analgesic), and reduce inflammation (anti-inflammatory). These actions are referred to as the three A's. The mechanism of action of aspirin and other NSAIDs is to inhibit the cyclooxygenase enzyme involved in the synthesis of prostaglandins from arachidonic acid. Prostaglandins are released from almost all cells in response to cell injury, and contribute to inflammation, pain, and fever. These chemicals may act at nerve ends and in the central nervous system. Another pathway in the metabolism of arachidonic acid involves the enzyme lipoxygenase, with subsequent formation of the leukotrienes. Many of these also are involved in the inflammatory response; however, none of the currently available cyclooxygenase inhibitors inhibit lipoxygenase. This may explain the lack of complete efficacy of the NSAIDs in treatment of inflammatory diseases.

The NSAIDs are analgesic and antipyretic at low doses. The anti-inflammatory actions of NSAIDs are seen only at the higher end of the dosage spectrum. These agents are used to treat inflammation of many causes. Although the inflammatory response is a defense mechanism, in some cases the inflammatory response is more damaging to tissues than the initiating injury factors.

The NSAIDs are comparable in efficacy, although not in potency. At equivalent anti-inflammatory doses, all are equally effective. However, the response of an individual patient to any particular drug is variable. This variability may be in effectiveness, side effects, or onset of response. Analgesic doses are inadequate for treatment of rheumatoid arthritis, gout, and osteoarthritis. However, as the dose is increased to that necessary for an anti-inflammatory response, the incidence of side effects increases, especially in the elderly. Anti-inflammatory doses of the NSAIDs are listed in Table 14–1.

ASPIRIN

Aspirin has been used for many decades and is a common household drug, found in most medicine cabinets. Its efficacy for many common musculoskeletal ailments is appreciated by many people. Aspirin is available in several forms. Although many people can take aspirin without any side effects, irritation of gastrointestinal mucosa may limit its use in some. Buffered aspirin (Bufferin) contains buffers that may decrease the gastric irritation. Enteric coated tablets prevent dissolution in the acid environment of the stomach (Ecotrin). This formulation is designed to prevent

TABLE 14–1.

Comparison of NSAID Potencies (Anti-inflammatory)

Drug	Total Daily Dose (mg)
Aspirin	4,000–6,000
Ibuprofen (Motrin, Advil, Nuprin)	1,600–3,200
Indomethacin (Indocin)	75–200
Meclofenamate (Ponstel, Meclomen)	300–400
Naproxen (Naprosyn, Anaprox)	500–1,000
Phenylbutazone (Butazolidin)	300–400
Piroxicam (Feldene)	10–20
Sulindac (Clinoril)	300–400
Tolmetin (Tolectin)	600–1,600
Flurbiprofen (Ansaid)	200–300

the irritation of the stomach that causes gastric ulcers. Timed release preparations are available (Zorprin) to extend the half-life of aspirin and to allow for overnight maintenance. Incomplete and variable absorption may result with either of the latter two preparations. The antipyretic-analgesic doses of aspirin are, for adults, 325 to 650 mg orally, every 4 hours. For children the dose is 65 mg/kg per day, given in 4 to 6 divided doses.

Acute aspirin overdose causes an initial stimulation directly on the respiratory center, causing hyperventilation and respiratory alkalosis. Continued high concentrations depress the respiratory center and renal function becomes impaired, causing a combination of respiratory acidosis and metabolic acidosis. Mild chronic aspirin toxicity resulting from anti-inflammatory dose therapy of arthritis, gout, or rheumatic fever may lead to "salicylism," with nausea, tinnitus, headache, hyperventilation, and central nervous system stimulation.

Aspirin is chemically acetylsalicylic acid. Sodium salicylate (Pabalate) is also available in oral form. Other salicylates are too toxic for systemic use. Salicylic acid (Compound W) is used topically as a keratolytic, for removal of warts and corns. Methyl salicylate (oil of wintergreen) is available for topical use as a counterirritant. It increases cutaneous blood flow and is used in treating painful muscles and joints. Its efficacy as a topical agent to treat systemic symptoms is doubtful. However, absorption can occur through the skin and lead to systemic poisoning.

Diflunisal (Dolobid) is another salicylate, but it is not antipyretic. It is, however, analgesic and anti-inflammatory, and is used in treatment of osteoarthritis. It also has less antiplatelet and gastrointestinal effects than aspirin. Diflunisal lacks the auditory side effect of aspirin.

NONASPIRIN NSAIDS

The nonaspirin NSAIDs also inhibit prostaglandin synthesis as their mechanism of action. The side effects are similar to those of aspirin. People hypersensitive to gastrointestinal irritation with aspirin generally have the same sensitivity to these agents. The most common adverse effects of NSAIDs are gastrointestinal and include heartburn, indigestion, nausea, vomiting, diarrhea, and constipation. Gastric ulcer disease may develop in 1% of patients during the first 6 to 12 months of treatment. Other potential serious side effects are neurotoxicity, hepatotoxicity (rare), and nephrotoxicity (more often seen in elderly patients with already compromised renal function, such as in heart failure, hypertension, and the nephrotic syndrome). Neurotoxicity may manifest as headache, changes in mental status, tinnitus, or hearing impairment. Aspirin has a greater propensity for 8th cranial nerve damage, while indomethacin (Indocin) is more likely to cause headache and changes in mental status. The central nervous system effects may be decreased if the drug is taken at bedtime.

The large number of drugs in this class, with newer ones added frequently, demonstrates the popularity of this type of pharmacologic intervention. The number of drugs also proves that the one "perfect" drug has not yet been developed. Generally, the NSAIDs produce similar therapeutic effects, if titrated to the maximum response. However, individuals may respond better to one agent than to another with respect to efficacy or tolerability.

Naproxen (Naprosyn, Anaprox) has been used for many years, and its pharmacologic profile is well studied. It is generally well tolerated, and dosage adjustment is generally not needed in the elderly or in those with only mild renal or hepatic impairment. Naproxen is available in two forms: as the pure drug (Naprosyn), and as the sodium salt of the drug (Anaprox). The sodium salt is more rapidly absorbed, thus producing an earlier and higher plasma concentration. This can be an advantage in relief of pain, but in chronic treatment, the two forms can be considered of equal efficacy. The potency ratio is 250 mg of naproxen being equal to 275 mg of naproxen sodium.

Piroxicam (Feldene), which is well tolerated, has a long half-life, allowing for once-a-day dosing. Sulindac (Clinoril) apparently spares the kidney and may be used in those at risk for nephrotoxicity. Phenylbutazone (Butazolidin) has serious adverse effects that limit its use, but it may be used acutely for inflammatory flare-ups. Aplastic anemia and agranulocytosis are the toxic effects resulting from its chronic use. If it is used for short (7- to 14-day) periods, serious adverse effects are not likely to develop. Indomethacin (Indocin) has the same indications and contraindications.

DRUG INTERACTIONS WITH THE NSAIDS

Aspirin and other NSAIDs have the propensity to interact with other drugs, even at analgesic/antipyretic doses. The NSAIDs generally have a high safety margin; however, very sick patients and the elderly may be more sensitive to development of adverse reactions. Because these agents are used so commonly, and generally without adverse effects, many people may not consider them as "drugs." This is especially true of the over-the-counter agents.

Certain patients using NSAIDs in combination with antihypertensive drugs, such as diuretics, beta blockers, angiotensin-converting enzyme inhibitors, and methyldopa (Aldomet), may show an increase in blood pressure. Indomethacin blocks the hypotensive response to propranolol (Inderal) and atenolol (Tenormin). Interestingly, naproxen and sulindac do not interfere with these beta blockers. Because they inhibit prostaglandin synthesis, NSAIDs may decrease the renal response to furosemide (Lasix) and other loop diuretics, which could potentially result in exacerbation of heart failure symptoms. Digoxin is eliminated by renal mechanisms. Concurrent administration of aspirin, indomethacin, or ibuprofen, which decrease renal clearance of digoxin, can lead to a toxic elevation of plasma levels of digoxin. Digoxin levels should be monitored during and after concurrent NSAID therapy. All the NSAIDs bind extensively to plasma proteins, and can cause displacement from the protein binding site, thus leading to toxic plasma levels of the drug. This interaction can be particularly significant with warfarin and the oral hypoglycemics. Aspirin probably should not be used in combination with warfarin. The other interaction between NSAIDs and warfarin relates to an increased propensity for bleeding problems, through inhibition of both platelet activity and coagulation factors. Aspirin and phenylbutazone (Butazolidin) increase the duration of action of the oral hypoglycemics. Tolmetin (Tolectin), however, in spite of its protein binding, does not interfere with concurrent warfarin or oral hypoglycemic administration.

The NSAIDs inhibit renal clearance of lithium, leading to lithium toxicity. Because of the very narrow therapeutic index for lithium, plasma concentrations need to be closely controlled to prevent toxicity, with readjustment of the lithium dose, if necessary. Meclofenamate (Ponstel, Meclomen) may cause diarrhea and should not be used by those concurrently taking oral gold medications, which also have the propensity to cause diarrhea. There are interactions between the NSAIDs and the antiepileptic agents. Phenylbutazone may increase phenytoin (Dilantin) levels. There is a multifaceted aspirin–valproic acid (Depakene) interaction that can lead to serious valproic acid toxicity.

PHYSICAL THERAPY NOTES

Because of the inhibition of platelet activity by the NSAIDs, people taking these drugs on a chronic basis have the potential for easy bruisability. Therefore, any trauma to soft tissue should be avoided. Thrombocytopenia, on the other hand, is a decreased number of platelets in the blood. This is a side effect of some drugs, although not of the NSAIDs. However, the effect on bruisability is the same, whether there is decreased function or a decreased number of platelets.

Many interactions are possible between aspirin and other drugs. A person taking aspirin along with other drugs should be on the alert for possible toxic reactions. Drug doses may need to be reduced.

Although aspirin and the NSAIDs have no effect on mental function, the presence or absence of pain and how a person deals with pain may have a tremendous influence on a person's mood. This can affect a person's interest in, and response to, physical therapy treatment.

LEARNING OBJECTIVES

1. Compare the differences and similarities between aspirin and the aspirin-like drugs with the nonaspirin analgesic, acetaminophen.
2. Know the side effects of long-term aspirin use.
3. Describe the types of drug-drug interactions between the NSAIDs and other drugs.

ADDITIONAL READINGS

1. Hochberg MC: NSAIDs: Mechanisms and pathways of action. *Hosp Pract* 1989; 24(Mar):185–198.
2. Hochberg MC: NSAIDs: Patterns of usage and side effects. *Hosp Pract* 1989; 24(May):167–174.
3. Karsh J: Adverse reactions and interactions with aspirin. *Drug Safety* 1990; 5:317–327.
4. Todd PA, Clissold SP: Naproxen, a reappraisal of its pharmacology, and therapeutic use in rheumatic diseases and pain states. *Drugs* 1990; 40:91–137.
5. Verbeeck RK: Pharmacokinetic drug interactions with nonsteroidal anti-inflammatory drugs. *Clin Pharmacokinet* 1990; 19:44–66.

Chapter 15

Glucocorticoids

Cortisol is a glucocorticoid hormone secreted by the adrenal cortex. Its secretion is regulated by hormones from the anterior pituitary gland and the hypothalamus. Corticotropin-releasing hormone (CRH) from the hypothalamus stimulates the release of adrenocorticotropic hormone (ACTH) from the anterior pituitary gland. In turn, ACTH stimulates the synthesis and the release of cortisol from the adrenal cortex. Cortisol has a negative feedback control on the release of both CRH and ACTH. Cortisol has important metabolic actions, and control of its secretion is in relation to the body's needs for cortisol, especially in times of stress. Another important aspect of the control of cortisol secretion relates to the ability of the central nervous system to override the hormonal control system. Secretion of cortisol exhibits a diurnal rhythm in people who are on normal schedules, with a peak early in the morning, then tapering off during the day, and beginning to rise again after midnight. The normal diurnal variation is related to sleep-wake cycles and is changed in shift workers, according to their sleep-wake schedules. The rescheduling of the cortisol rhythm following changes in sleep-wake cycles associated with crossing several time zones is, in part, the cause of "jet lag."

Metabolic actions of cortisol are more of a "permissive" nature, in that other hormones exert their actions in the presence of cortisol. The actions of cortisol are best described in comparing hypocortisolism and hypercortisolism. In tissues other than the liver, cortisol has actions that result in decreased uptake and utilization of glucose, increased lipolysis, and increased proteolysis. In the liver, cortisol increases protein synthesis, increases glycogen synthesis and storage, and increases gluconeogenesis. Cortisol also increases fat deposition in abdominal adipose tissue. Cortisol is important in maintenance of normal skeletal muscle function. Deviations from the normal concentration, either increases or decreases, cause skeletal muscle weakness.

Clinically, the most important use of glucocorticoids is for their anti-inflammatory actions. The relationship of these actions to normal physiology is not clear.

PHARMACOLOGIC USES OF GLUCOCORTICOIDS

Cortisol is the naturally occurring glucocorticoid, and although used in certain situations, it also has aldosterone-like or mineralocorticoid activity. The synthetic glucocorticoids have decreased, or are void of, mineralocorticoid activity. However, separation of the two glucocorticoid actions, metabolic and anti-inflammatory, has not yet been possible. All glucocorticoids thus have significant metabolic activity.

Glucocorticoids are often used in treatment of inflammatory or immune diseases, such as rheumatoid arthritis, bronchial asthma, collagen diseases, allergic conditions, and inflammatory eye conditions. The use of glucocorticoids in inflammatory and immune disorders is not curative. In these diseases, the inflammatory response and subsequent immune complex formation may be more damaging than the disease itself. It is the inflammatory and immune responses that are inhibited, but not the cause of the response. The mechanism of anti-inflammatory action of cortisol is not completely understood, but it possibly controls the synthesis of phospholipase inhibitory proteins, such as lipocortin. Lipocortin is thought to inhibit phospholipase in the cell membrane and thus synthesis of products of both the lipoxygenase and the cyclooxygenase pathways. Thus, glucocorticoids inhibit the synthesis of leukotrienes and the prostanoids, which are mediators of the inflammatory response. The inhibition of lipoxygenase in addition to inhibition of cyclooxygenase by glucocorticoids possibly explains their greater efficacy in inflammatory diseases than the nonsteroidal anti-inflammatory drugs (NSAIDs) (see Fig 14–1).

Because of the metabolic derangements apparent with chronic glucocorticoid use, these drugs should not be considered benign. A short course of treatment, even with a relatively high dose, especially in life-threatening situations, is generally of no basis for concern. In chronic treatment of inflammatory conditions, however, the dose should be appropriate to maintain the symptoms within tolerable limits. Disability is a reason for use of glucocorticoids; however, complete relief of symptoms is not sought.

The major difference among the synthetic glucocorticoids relates to the duration of action (Table 15–1). In order to avoid some adverse effects of chronic use, alternate-day therapy (ADT) may be attempted. In this situation, a short-acting or intermediate acting preparation is given in the morning, at the time of the normal cortisol peak. The drug is then metabolized during the day, and thus does not inhibit the cortisol peak on the 2nd day, when no drug is given. On the 3rd day, a second dose of the short-acting preparation is given. This more likely will not result in adrenal suppression, and in many cases will control the inflammatory aspects of the disease. If ADT does not sufficiently suppress symptoms, administration in the morning is preferred to evening administration, to coincide with the normal diurnal peak.

Prolonged (more than a few weeks) treatment with high doses of gluco-

TABLE 15–1.

Glucocorticoid Preparations

Short acting (biologic half-life, 8–12 hr)	
Cortisol	(Cortef, Hydrocortone)
Cortisone	(Cortone)
Intermediate acting (biologic half-life, 12–36 hr)	
Prednisone	(Deltasone, Orasone, Meticorten)
Prednisolone	(Delta Cortef, Cortolone)
6-Methylprednisolone	(Medrol)
Triamcinolone	(Aristocort)
Long acting (biologic half-life, 36–72 hr)	
Paramethasone	(Haldrone)
Betamethasone	(Celestone)
Dexamethasone	(Decadron)

corticoids always produces some degree of adrenal cortex suppression. For this reason, after chronic therapy, a person is slowly withdrawn from the drug. Too rapid of a withdrawal may produce signs and symptoms of adrenal insufficiency, which may be life-threatening. The time needed for appropriate withdrawal relates to the degree of suppression. Tapered withdrawal from severe suppression can take weeks to months before the anterior pituitary-adrenal cortex axis becomes fully functional. Symptoms of adrenal insufficiency are fever, myalgia, arthralgia, and malaise.

The decision for chronic glucocorticoid administration must balance possible, and probable, adverse effects of the drug vs. the degree of functional impairment and disability without using the drug. Because of the metabolic derangements induced with chronic glucocorticoid use, these drugs should not be considered as benign. Glucocorticoids can be administered orally, parenterally, and topically. Topical use of glucocorticoids to treat dermatologic conditions may not produce systemic side effects. Dermatologic conditions amenable to glucocorticoid treatment are allergic skin conditions, psoriasis, seborrheic dermatitis, and erythema multiforma. However, even topical administration can cause systemic effects with adrenal suppression if significant absorption occurs. Systemic side effects are more likely to occur if a large surface area is treated and if an occlusive plastic wrap is used. Inflammatory eye conditions may be treated with topical glucocorticoids. A serious adverse effect is increased intraocular pressure. This may not be reversible, so intraocular pressure should be monitored during treatment.

Glucocorticoids may be used to treat rheumatoid arthritis, when the disease is progressive and disability is not controlled by NSAIDs, gold, and other agents. Chronic glucocorticoid treatment carries the risk of osteoporosis. This is especially a concern in those at high risk for osteoporosis, such as postmenopausal women and elderly men. The NSAIDs may be used concurrently with glucocorticoids. However, there is some concern for development of peptic ulcer with the use of both of these drugs. If only one or a few joints are involved, intra-articular injection may be used to eliminate systemic effects. However, repeated intra-articular injection can cause destruction of the joint.

The use of systemic glucocorticoids in asthma should be reserved for severe cases that do not respond to other methods of treatment and for status asthmaticus. Currently, the use of inhaled glucocorticoids in children is promoted by some clinicians because of the behavioral problems associated with theophylline. If administered properly using an inhaler, there is little likelihood for systemic absorption of glucocorticoids. However, because of the possibility for growth retardation in children, careful monitoring of systemic effects is important.

Glucocorticoids depress all aspects of the immune system. For this reason the glucocorticoids are frequently used in treatment of autoimmune diseases. Autoimmune diseases are an example of the function of the immune system acting against one's own tissues, instead of against foreign bodies. During development there is a "filtering" of immune cells that would react against one's cells, the recognition of "self" vs. "nonself." With autoimmune diseases, a situation occurs such that the immune cells recognize "self" as "nonself."

ADVERSE EFFECTS

Adverse effects from chronic glucocorticoid use are multiple and affect many body systems. Fluid and electrolyte disturbances may occur with development of hypertension, depending on the mineralocorticoid activity of the specific drug. Metabolic alterations lead to a redistribution of body fat to the torso (centripetal obesity), face (moon face), and back of the neck (buffalo hump). There is also the possibility of development of hyperglycemia, similar to diabetes mellitus because glucocorticoids counteract the actions of insulin. Effects of glucocorticoids on protein synthesis can lead to muscle wasting and muscle weakness, termed "steroid myopathy." This weakness is especially prevalent in the proximal limb muscles, and may not be reversible after discontinuation of the drug. Proliferation of fibroblasts and deposition of collagen are decreased with chronic glucocorticoid treatment and are responsible for decreased scar formation. This alteration in collagen formation is responsible also for a loss of connective tissue and development of striae. Central nervous system effects from chronic use of glucocorticoids can lead to behavioral disturbances, from nervousness and changes in mood to psychoses. Glucocorticoids can promote development and spread of infection, and delay healing. The presence of an infection in a person who is taking glucocorticoids may not be a reason to discontinue the glucocorticoid, if appropriate anti-infective therapy is also administered. Glucocorticoids inhibit the growth plate in long bones and can cause growth retardation in children. This limits their chronic systemic use in this age group. Chronic use of glucocorticoids can hasten the processes involved in osteoporosis and promote vertebral compression fractures. This is of particular concern in the elderly. Capillary fragility is increased with chronic use of the glucocorticoids, and is responsible for easy bruisability in those patients who have been taking glucocorticoids on a chronic basis.

The cellular actions initiated by the glucocorticoids continue much longer than the period during which the drug remains in the plasma. This is referred to as the drug's biological half-life.

PHYSIOLOGIC USE OF GLUCOCORTICOIDS

Glucocorticoids are used for replacement therapy in adrenal insufficiency, which is considered physiologic replacement. The doses used are to simulate the endogenous glucocorticoid production. Thus, the adverse effects mentioned earlier do not occur. Maintenance of the diurnal rhythm of blood levels of glucocorticoids is produced by administration of two thirds of the total daily dose in the morning and one third of the dose in the evening.

PHYSICAL THERAPY NOTES

Of interest to physical therapists is the recent report on the use of methylprednisolone in treatment of acute spinal cord injury. The inflammatory response to the injury appears to be detrimental to nerve viability. Immediate treatment with glucocorticoids apparently inhibits the inflammatory response, allowing for nerve preservation. The mechanisms behind tissue damage secondary to the inflammatory response are an area of intense scientific investigation.

The use of glucocorticoids in treatment of asthma is discussed in Chapter 18. Because of the growth inhibitory actions of glucocorticoids, their chronic use in children has been discouraged. However, inhalation therapy with the drugs appears to be effective and without systemic side effects.

The major symptoms of toxicity seen with chronic glucocorticoid use are easy bruisability, poor wound healing, proximal muscle weakness, and osteoporosis. All of these are probably related, in part, to decreased protein synthesis. A possible toxic reaction to chronic use of glucocorticoids is development of a psychosis. This is more likely with high doses, and in the elderly.

LEARNING OBJECTIVES

1. Understand the normal control mechanisms of glucocorticoid secretion, including negative feedback and the diurnal rhythm.
2. Know the drawbacks of glucocorticoid therapy in chronic inflammatory diseases and why alternate-day therapy may alleviate some side effects.
3. List the methods of administration of glucocorticoids and why topical administration can cause systemic effects.
4. Explain the adverse effects which are possible with chronic glucocorticoid use.

ADDITIONAL READINGS

1. Bracken MB, Shepard MJ, Collins WF, et al: A randomized, controlled trial of methyl-prednisolone or naloxone in the treatment of acute spinal-cord injury. *N Engl J Med* 1990; 322:1405–1411.
2. DiRosa M, Calignano A, Carnucio R, et al: Multiple control of inflammation by glucocorticoids. *Agents Actions* 1985; 17:284–289.
3. Flower RJ: Lipocortin and the mechanisms of action of the glucocorticoids. *Br J Pharmacol* 1988; 94:987–1015.

Chapter 16

Drugs Used in Treatment of Arthritic Diseases

RHEUMATOID ARTHRITIS

Rheumatoid arthritis is a chronic, inflammatory disease of unknown cause. It involves an activation of cellular inflammatory and immune responses in a genetically susceptible individual. There may be many different stimuli which can activate the immune response. One proposed causative factor is a virus that either activates the immune response or cross-reacts with host tissue. Autoimmunity has a major role in progression of the disease, but data supporting autoimmunity as the initial cause of rheumatoid arthritis are less firm. Rheumatoid arthritis is characterized by a persistent inflammatory synovitis, which usually involves peripheral joints in a symmetrical distribution. Locally produced immune complexes activate complement. Activated complement can activate leukocytes, which then ingest immune complexes and release inflammatory mediators, such as superoxide, adding to the inflammatory response. This is a positive-feedback cycle, with continuing activation of leukocytes and release of chemical mediators of inflammation. Manifestations of the chronic inflammation are hyperplasia and hypertrophy of synovial lining cells. The infiltrating cell is the helper T cell, which produces a variety of inflammatory chemicals, such as interleukin-2, chemotactic factors, and B cell activation. The potential of the chronic synovial inflammation to cause cartilage destruction and bone erosion and subsequently joint deformities is a hallmark of this disease. The disease can follow a variable course, with remissions and exacerbations, but it is generally of a progressive nature. A clear and permanent remission is rare. There seems to be a genetic predisposition to rheumatoid arthritis. There is also a genetic predisposition of development of toxic reactions to drugs used to treat the disease, especially gold and penicillamine.

The onset of symptoms is usually gradual, with fatigue, anorexia, generalized weakness and vague musculoskeletal symptoms appearing before the synovitis. Extraarticular

TABLE 16–1.

Diagnostic Criteria* for Rheumatoid Arthritis

1. Morning stiffness
2. Arthritis of three or more joint areas
3. Arthritis of hand joints
4. Symmetric arthritis
5. Rheumatoid nodules
6. Serum rheumatoid factor
7. Radiologic changes typical of rheumatoid arthritis

*A person is classified as having rheumatoid arthritis if meeting at least four of these seven criteria. Criteria 1 through 4 must have been present for at least 6 weeks.

manifestations such as rheumatoid nodules appear on periarticular structures. Skeletal muscular weakness and atrophy contribute to the debilitating aspects of the disease. Rheumatoid vasculitis, polyneuropathy, cutaneous ulceration, and necrosis may also be present. Pleuropulmonary manifestations such as pleural disease, pneumonitis, and fibrosis may be evident. There also may be an asymptomatic pericarditis.

The metacarpophalangeal joints, proximal interphalangeal joints, and wrists are the first joints to become symptomatic. Although rheumatoid arthritis is a symmetrical disease, interestingly in patients with unilateral paresis, there is rarely inflammatory synovitis in the paralyzed limb, if arthritis develops subsequently. This demonstrates the requirement for an intact neuromuscular unit in the development of rheumatoid arthritis. However, at present nothing is understood about this involvement.

No laboratory tests are specific for the diagnosis of rheumatoid arthritis. Rheumatoid factors, which are circulating IgM antibodies against IgG molecules, are present in high titer, but are not specific for rheumatoid arthritis, in that they increase with increasing age. Diagnosis is based on clinical criteria. The American Rheumatism Association has defined criteria for the diagnosis of rheumatoid arthritis (Table 16–1).

Because the cause of rheumatoid arthritis is unknown, the therapy is aimed at alleviating symptoms. None of the therapies, however, is curative. Most pharmacologic treatments involve nonspecific suppression of the inflammatory process. This is a chronic disease with periods of apparent remissions followed by flares of activity. Treatment of the arthritic patient involves a multidisciplinary approach. Effective therapy must be instituted early to prevent irreversible loss of articular cartilage. Physical therapy includes rest of the involved joints during acute flare-ups to minimize damage, splinting to prevent deforming contractures from developing and to reduce motion of inflamed joints, and exercise of the involved joints during non-flare-ups to maintain range of motion and muscle strength without exacerbating joint inflammation. The inflamed joint is especially vulnerable to the effects of motion. In joints with effusions, exercise may increase intra-articular pressures sufficient to decrease synovial blood flow and cause ischemia and, eventually, tissue necrosis. When joints develop effusions, they are normally flexed 5° to 20°, because full extension is too painful. An increased level of activity during periods of remission may help reduce bone loss. Exercise of weight-bearing joints is one of the best known methods to enhance bone mineral content. Very little

TABLE 16–2.

Pharmacologic Management of Rheumatoid Arthritis

Drug	Advantages	Disadvantages
First line		
Aspirin	Analgesic, anti-inflammatory	Gastrointestinal symptoms, does not modify disease
Nonaspirin NSAIDs	Fewer gastrointestinal symptoms	Does not modify disease
Second line		
Gold	Disease modifying	Cytopenias
Hydroxychloroquine	Well-tolerated, inexpensive	Optical toxicity; moderate efficacy
Penicillamine	High efficacy	May induce autoimmune disease; cytopenias
Third line		
Azathioprine	Well-tolerated, high efficacy	Altered liver function; cytopenias
Methotrexate	Weekly dose regimen	Cytopenias
Glucocorticoids	Low doses well tolerated	At high doses: peptic ulcer, adrenal suppression, Cushing's syndrome

gross destruction of articular cartilage is necessary before its normal function is weakened to the point that progressive disintegration occurs in response to the exercise of weight-bearing joints or to muscular contractions during normal activities of daily living. Orthotic devices may be necessary to support and align deformed joints, to reduce pain, and to allow for increased function.

Pharmacologic treatment includes aspirin or other nonsteroidal anti-inflammatory drugs (NSAIDs), steroidal anti-inflammatory agents, or disease-modifying agents. Advantages and disadvantages of the various drugs are listed in Table 16–2. Aspirin and other NSAIDs are the foundation of drug therapy in rheumatoid arthritis. However, they are not thought to have much effect on the underlying disease process itself. The slow-acting or disease-modifying drugs are used in those patients who have inadequate response to the NSAIDs. About half the patients with rheumatoid arthritis will progress to this category. In severe cases, surgery may be indicated. It is most successful in hip and knee replacement.

Nonsteroidal Anti-inflammatory Agents

Anti-inflammatory doses of aspirin and other NSAIDs are well tolerated by many patients without gastric distress, particularly when enteric coated preparations are used. Tinnitus, which is relatively harmless, indicates therapeutic levels for an anti-inflammatory response. The use of NSAIDs is to suppress the inflammatory process in hopes of ameliorating symptoms and preventing progressive damage to articular structures. In treatment of rheumatoid arthritis, none of the NSAIDs is more effective than aspirin, but other drugs may have a lower incidence of gastrointestinal side effects. The enteric coated preparations may reduce the gastrointestinal side effects; however, bioavailability of the drug may be compromised. Patients who do not respond to one NSAID may respond to another. For a more complete discussion of the NSAIDs, see Chapter 14.

Steroidal Anti-inflammatory Agents

Glucocorticoids are effective treatment for rheumatoid arthritis. However, because of the chronic nature of this disease and the toxicity associated with chronic use of glucocorticoids, their use is reserved for treatment of progressive disability that is not controlled by NSAIDs, gold, and other agents. A more complete discussion of glucocorticoids is in Chapter 15.

Slow-Acting or Disease-Modifying Agents

The slow-acting agents are also referred to as disease-modifying agents, reflecting the optimism that these agents really do alter the course of the disease. These drugs are reserved for those with rapidly progressive disease or who fail to respond adequately to the NSAIDs. Time to onset of therapeutic response with these agents may be up to several months. Treatment should continue for up to 6 months before a treatment failure is considered. With most of the slow-acting drugs, there is a loss of therapeutic effectiveness occurring with time (secondary failure). Lack of response to one drug does not predict response to another. The NSAIDs should be continued during this early time, to allow at least some protection. All of these agents are associated with toxicity. Part of the expense associated with their use is laboratory monitoring for toxic reactions.

Gold Therapy (Chrysotherapy)

The gold compounds are thought to retard disease progression by inhibiting lysosomal enzymes and decreasing phagocytic activity of macrophages, thus reducing the inflammatory response. Three months of treatment may be necessary before an improvement is noticed. Gold treatment is available in both oral and parenteral (intramuscular) forms. Oral gold, auranofin (Ridaura), is not as effective as the parenteral form, but it is less toxic. More frequent side effects are related to the gastrointestinal tract, with loose stools and diarrhea. The diarrhea may be controlled by bismuth subsalicylate (Pepto-Bismol). Other adverse effects, such as rashes, skin lesions, blood dyscrasias, and proteinuria are less common than with parenteral therapy. However, regular laboratory monitoring is required.

Parenteral gold therapy, aurothioglucose (Solganal) or sodium thiomalate, gold (Myochrysine), given by intramuscular injection, from weekly to monthly, depending on the state of the disease. Toxicity is mainly in the form of blood dyscrasias, such as thrombocytopenia or granulocytopenia, and renal toxicity, seen as proteinuria. Most side effects occur within the first 6 months of treatment. In the absence of toxicity, these agents may be given as long as beneficial responses are seen.

Antimalarials

Chloroquine and hydroxychloroquine (Plaquenil) are antimalarial drugs that are also effective in treatment of rheumatoid arthritis. They appear to act by suppressing formation of the antigens involved in the hypersensitivity reactions that are responsible for collagen disease processes. The antimalarials also are used in treatment of systemic lupus erythematosus, another multisystem disease involving overstimulation of the immune system. Side effects are fairly rare and mainly involve the gastrointestinal tract. With long-term use there may be pigment changes affecting hair, skin, and mucous membranes, although this is uncommon. Their serious toxicity, although uncommon, relates to the drug being deposited in the eye, leading to blindness. These agents are fairly well tolerated, and are the least toxic, especially hydroxychloroquine. They are also the least expensive. Toxicity testing involves twice a year ophthalmic examinations to check for drug accumulation in the retina.

Penicillamine

Penicillamine (Cuprimine, Depen) has the slowest onset of action of the slow-acting drugs. The most common side effects are gastrointestinal, particularly nausea and dysgeusia (loss of taste). The loss of the sense of taste may be very disconcerting to the patient, but it is usually transient, and tolerance develops in about a month or two. Skin rashes are less common than with parenteral gold. Major toxicity is seen as the cytopenias, nephrotoxicity and induction of autoimmune diseases, such as systemic lupus erythematosus, myasthenia gravis, and polymyositis. Again, complete blood counts and urinalysis are necessary to monitor for toxicity.

Azathioprine

Azathioprine (Imuran) is approved for treatment of rheumatoid arthritis that has been unresponsive to conventional therapy. This agent is both an antimetabolite and an immunosuppressant. It depresses actively replicating helper T cells and, presumably, B cell proliferation. It is one of the more effective of the slow-acting agents and is better tolerated than parenteral gold or penicillamine. The most common side effects are nausea and other gastrointestinal symptoms, abnormalities in liver function, and leukopenia. Monthly blood counts and liver function tests are needed to monitor for toxicity. There is no known renal toxicity. The suspicion that it may be oncogenic has limited its widespread use; however, there is no clear correlation to date between azathioprine and oncogenesis.

Methotrexate

Methotrexate is another cytotoxic-immunosuppressant agent that has been used in treatment of cancer. It has recently been approved by the U.S. Food and Drug Administration (FDA) for treatment of rheumatoid arthritis that has not responded to at least one other slow-acting agent. This drug has a more rapid onset of action than the other slow-acting agents. The therapeutic effect is seen in 3 to 6 weeks. This agent is possibly anti-inflammatory, whereas the other slow-acting agents are not. It also has a longer duration of response in that secondary failures are less likely to occur. The immediate side effects are stomatitis, nausea, vomiting, and transient disturbances in liver function. Switching from the oral to the intramuscular preparation may partially prevent these side effects. In fact, the parenteral form is cheaper than the oral, provided it can be administered at home. Cytotoxic and immunosuppressive effects are generally not seen at the doses used in the treatment of rheumatoid arthritis. The serious adverse effects are the cytopenias, cirrhosis, and an acute pneumonia-like syndrome. Routine blood counts and liver function tests are necessary to monitor for toxicity. This agent is contraindicated in patients with underlying lung diseases.

Sulfasalazine

Sulfasalazine, although not approved by the FDA for treatment of rheumatoid arthritis, has been used experimentally for this indication. Side effects are mainly gastrointestinal, with nausea, abdominal pain, and anorexia, the most common. It appears to have a better safety profile than parenteral gold, with a low incidence of hepatic toxicity and leukopenia. However, liver function and blood counts should still be done every 2 to 3 months.

OSTEOARTHRITIS

Osteoarthritis, or degenerative joint disease, is the most common of the arthropathies. Its cause is unknown. It is thought to be associated with aging, but it may be a genetic disorder, associated with faulty collagen synthesis. It more frequently involves weight-bearing or frequently used joints. There is a loss of articular cartilage and remodeling of subchondral bone. Hypertrophic new bone develops beyond the joint margins, leading to nodes.

Osteoarthritis can be differentiated from rheumatoid arthritis by the joints involved and the types of joint deformities. In osteoarthritis, the distal interphalangeal (DIP) and proximal interphalangeal (PIP) joints are commonly involved, with evidence of wrist disease. In rheumatoid arthritis, on the other hand, the metacarpophalangeal, PIP, and wrist joints are commonly involved; however, the DIP joints are rarely involved. In osteoarthritis the cervical and lumbar spine may be involved, but the lumbar spine is rarely involved in rheumatoid arthritis. There are nodular involvements in osteoarthritis, which are not seen in rheumatoid arthritis. Heberden's nodes are located on the DIP joint and Bouchard's nodes are on the PIP. The joint deformities and nodes give a flexed and lateral deviation of the fingers.

The goals of treatment are to decrease pain and to maintain range of motion and function, without incurring further damage. Pharmacologic treatment is with aspirin and other NSAIDs, using anti-inflammatory doses at times of acute flare-ups.

GOUT

Gout is an inflammatory disease characterized by uric acid crystals in joint fluid and soft tissues. The first metatarsophalangeal joint is frequently involved. Podagra is the term used to indicate a painful and swollen great toe. The hallmark of the disease is hyperuricemia. Hyperuricemia results when the metabolic production of uric acid is greater than its renal excretion. This may be due to overproduction, underexcretion, or a combination of both. Crystals develop when the uric acid concentration is above levels where the urate can remain in solution. Precipitation of urate crystals depends on the level and duration of hyperuricemia. Urate crystals form in the synovial fluid and this crystallization activates an inflammatory response. Activated leukocytes phagocytose the crystals. Urate crystals can also precipitate around joints, forming tophi, or in other soft tissues, such as the kidney. This latter can lead to kidney damage. With hyperuricemia there is also the possibility of forming urate-containing kidney stones (nephrolithiasis).

Although gout is a chronic disease, its course is variable. Acute attacks are very painful, with one or more joints involved. An acute attack may last from days to weeks, interspersed with symptom-free times, which may last up to several years.

The goals of treatment are to terminate an acute attack and to prevent subsequent attacks. Drugs used in treatment of gout are either anti-inflammatory, prevent uric acid reabsorption from renal tubules, or prevent uric acid formation. Colchicine is the agent most commonly used to terminate an acute attack and is most effective if therapy is begun soon after the onset of symptoms. Colchicine is anti-inflammatory, specifically in gouty arthritis. However, it is not analgesic. Colchicine is administered at 1 mg every 2 hours until symptoms abate or side effects limit its use.

Indomethacin (Indocin) may be used if the side effects of colchicine are not tolerable. Even though indomethacin has its attendant side effects, they seem better tolerated than those of colchicine, especially if treatment is limited to 3 to 5 days. Indomethacin is generally more effective than colchicine if initiation of therapy has been prolonged after onset of symptoms.

Prevention of recurrent attacks includes dietary changes, with weight reduction in obese patients, avoidance of heavy alcohol intake, and avoidance of foods rich in purines, such as organ meats. Colchicine can be used on a chronic basis in smaller doses than are used to treat an acute attack, at 1 to 2 mg/day. Gastrointestinal problems, such as nausea, vomiting, diarrhea, and abdominal pain can be severe, especially in the elderly.

Antihyperuricemic drugs that either decrease production or increase excretion of uric acid can also be used. Uric acid is formed by the oxidation of hypoxanthine to xanthine and the further oxidation of xanthine to uric acid. These reactions are catalyzed by the enzyme xanthine oxidase. Allopurinol (Zyloprim) is a specific inhibitor of this enzyme. There are few side effects, other than gastrointestinal distress, from its chronic use. This is rarely sufficient for discontinuance of the drug. Allopurinol is administered at 300 mg, once a day.

Probenecid (Benemid, Probalan) decreases renal absorption of uric acid and thus increases uric acid excretion in urine. This may lead to formation of urate kidney stones in susceptible individuals. Gastrointestinal complaints may be sufficient to discontinue this drug. The usual dose of probenecid in treatment of gout is 250 to 500 mg, twice daily. Probenecid is completely absorbed after oral administration and is excreted by renal mechanisms. Sulfinpyrazone (Anturane, Aprazone) also reduces renal reabsorption of uric acid and increases urinary excretion. Its action is additive to that of probenecid. The usual dose of sulfinpyrazone in treatment of gout is 200 to 800 mg/day in three or four divided doses. Sulfinpyrazone may cause gastric distress, but this can be decreased if the drug is taken with meals. Aspirin blocks the uricosuric action of probenecid and sulfinpyrazone, so it should not be used concurrently.

PHYSICAL THERAPY NOTES

Physical therapy is very important in the total management of the arthritic patient. The overall goal of therapy is to maintain function and to prevent further deterioration of functional level, without causing undue injury. This involves alternating between active treatment, such as exercise, and passive treatment, with rest and splinting, as the course of the disease varies. Although maintenance of joint range of motion is a goal of therapy, joint motion during an acute episode of inflammation and swelling may cause tissue damage. However, bed rest during the active phase of rheumatoid arthritis, if prolonged, can cause deconditioning, with its attendant problems.

Anti-inflammatory doses of NSAIDs are necessary for treatment of arthritis. Analgesic doses are insufficient. There is considerable individual variation in efficacy and toxicity in response to the different NSAIDs. If one agent is not well tolerated or effective, another agent should be substituted.

LEARNING OBJECTIVES

1. Understand the pathophysiology of arthritis, including the inflammatory-immune responses.
2. Describe the actions of the various classes of drugs used to treat the arthritides, such as NSAIDs, glucocorticoids, gold, and antimetabolites.
3. Describe the adverse effects associated with each of the groups of drugs (NSAIDs, glucocorticoids, gold, antimetabolites, and others).

ADDITIONAL READINGS

1. Arnett FC, Edworthy SM, Bloch DA, et al: The American Rheumatism Association 1987 revised criteria for the classification of rheumatoid arthritis. *Arthritis Rheum* 1988; 31:315–324.
2. Arnold M, Schrieber L, Brooks P: Immunosuppressive drugs and corticosteroids in the treatment of rheumatoid arthritis. *Drugs* 1988; 36:340–363.
3. Hardin JG: Rheumatoid arthritis therapy: The slow-acting agents. *Hosp Pract* 1989; 24(June):163–178.
4. Harris ED: Rheumatoid arthritis. *N Engl J Med* 1990; 322:1277–1289.
5. Marino C, McDonald E, Desai C, et al: Management of acute gout: Current role of colchicine and other treatment regimens. *Hosp Formul* 1990; 25:979–982.
6. Merry P, Winyard PG, Morris CJ, et al: Oxygen free radicals, inflammation, and synovitis: The current status. *Ann Rheum Dis* 1989; 48:864–870.
7. Wolfe CS, Hughes GRV: The optimum management of arthropathies. *Drugs* 1988; 36:370–381.

Chapter 17

Drugs Used in Treatment of Neuromuscular Immune/ Inflammatory Diseases

This chapter provides a discussion of several neuromuscular diseases that have in common muscular weakness as their chief complaint and immune/inflammatory processes as their proposed cause.

MYASTHENIA GRAVIS

Myasthenia gravis is a neuromuscular disease characterized by weakness and marked fatigability of skeletal muscle. Exacerbations and partial remissions occur frequently. Sustained remissions of greater than 2 years are, however, rare. Myasthenia gravis appears to be an acquired autoimmune response to the nicotinic II acetylcholine receptor at the neuromuscular junction, resulting from an interplay of both genetic and environmental factors. The antibodies reduce the number of receptors available at the postsynaptic membrane by increasing receptor degradation. There is, thus, a more rapid turnover of receptors. In healthy individuals the acetylcholine receptor usually persists for about a week; in myasthenia gravis, the receptors remain only about a day. The extraocular and bulbar muscles are most commonly affected. The order of frequency of muscle involvement is facial muscles, neck, limb girdles, distal limbs, and, finally, trunk muscles. The disease may involve external ocular muscles selectively. The initial skeletal muscle response to electrical stimulation may be normal, but the response diminishes rapidly. It is difficult for the patient to maintain voluntary muscular activity for more than brief period. Muscle strength is decreased with effort and improves with rest.

Pharmacologic Treatment

Pharmacologic treatment of myasthenia gravis involves two avenues of treatment. The first is the use of anticholinesterase drugs that inhibit breakdown of acetylcholine, so the neurotransmitter remains at the motor end plate longer. These drugs have no effect on the underlying disease. The second approach to treatment of myasthenia gravis is aimed at the immunologic aspects of the disease. This includes the use of glucocorticoids and immunosuppressives, and other treatments, such as thymectomy and plasmapheresis.

Cholinesterase Inhibitors

The anticholinsterase drugs inhibit acetylcholinesterase at the motor end plate and thus inhibit the degradation of acetylcholine. This allows acetylcholine to remain in the neuromuscular junction for a longer time and increases interactions between acetylcholine and its nicotinic II receptor. The goal of therapy is to strive for maximal therapeutic effect with minimal side effects. With inhibition of acetylcholinesterase the side effects are attributable to increased acetylcholine availability in other cholinergic sites, especially muscarinic.

The more commonly used drugs are pyridostigmine bromide (Mestinon) and neostigmine (Prostigmin). Pyridostigmine is used more frequently because it has fewer muscarinic side effects and a more prolonged duration of action. It is not well absorbed from the intestinal tract after oral administration, so its bioavailability is variable. Concurrent administration of bulk laxatives, such as methylcellulose, almost completely inhibit absorption. Pyridostigmine has a duration of action of 3 to 6 hours, but is also available in a slow-release formulation that can provide overnight coverage.

Cholinergic crisis is due to an excess of the anticholinesterase agent. It is characterized by weakness from generalized depolarization of the motor end plate and overstimulation of muscarinic receptors (parasympathetic postganglionics). Signs and symptoms are abdominal cramps, vomiting, diarrhea, miosis, increased glandular secretions and bradycardia.

Myasthenic crisis, on the other hand, is due to refractoriness to the drug. It is characterized by progressive weakness but no muscarinic effects. In this situation, other treatments are attempted. These include mere support of organ systems, especially respiratory, or more drastic measures such as alternate-day therapy with corticosteroids, thymectomy, immunosuppressants, or plasmapheresis. The myasthenic crisis may be transient, and after a period of time, the anticholinesterases may be effective again. The refractoriness is an exacerbation of the disease, the cause of which is not known.

Glucocorticoids

Glucocorticoids are used in treatment of those patients who have not responded well to the anticholinesterase drugs. Ocular myasthenia responds poorly to the anticholinesterase drugs and also to thymectomy. Chronic use of glucocorticoids is warranted, even with the attendant side effects, to decrease the disability. The lowest dose possible is used to decrease the toxicity of chronic glucocorticoid use. Two to 3 weeks of treatment are usually necessary before beneficial effects are seen. Alternate-day therapy may be effective, and should be attempted. A combination of a glucocorticoid with an anticholinesterase may allow for lower doses of each, and a reduction in side effects.

Azathioprine

The immunosuppressive drug azathioprine (Imuran) may be effective in treatment of myasthenia gravis. It reduces levels of the acetylcholine receptor antibody and improves clinical status. Clinical improvement may take 6 to 12 weeks of treatment. This drug can, however, cause bone marrow suppression, so blood cell monitoring is required.

Other Treatments

Plasmapheresis provides dramatic, but short-lived, improvement in clinical status. Thymectomy may allow for complete remission; however, several years may elapse before clinical benefits become apparent.

IDIOPATHIC INFLAMMATORY MYOPATHIES

Dermatomyositis and polymyositis are characterized by muscle weakness associated with inflammatory infiltrates in the muscle. Dermatomyositis also includes a characteristic dark-colored rash on the face, in a butterfly pattern over the bridge of the nose and cheeks, and on the eyelids, torso, and other sites. Dermatomyositis, with its proximal muscular weakness associated with the characteristic skin rash, is fairly easy to diagnose. Polymyositis, without the skin involvement, is more difficult to diagnose. These muscular disorders are frequently associated with connective tissue disorders such as systemic lupus erythematosus or rheumatoid arthritis, suggesting a common autoimmune etiology. The dominant features are muscular weakness of the limb girdle and proximal muscles. An afflicted person has difficulty getting out of a chair. The distal muscles are generally spared, as are the ocular muscles. Muscle atrophy is rare. Tendon reflexes are not decreased. In fact, they may be increased.

Pharmacologic Treatment

A glucocorticoid, especially prednisone, is the accepted treatment; however, there are no controlled studies to prove this. Initially, 60 to 100 mg/day for adults is administered until significant improvement is seen, which may require 3 months. Then the dose is reduced, or alternate-day therapy is attempted, to find a maintenance dose. If glucocorticoids do not provide satisfactory improvement, the cytotoxic drugs, such as azathioprine or methotrexate, may be used.

An adverse effect of long-term glucocorticoid use is myopathy. After the inflammatory myopathy has been stabilized, development of muscular weakness may be due to steroid-induced myopathy or to a relapse in the disease. To treat this, the glucocorticoid dose is reduced. If the weakness is due to glucocorticoid toxicity, the clinical situation will improve. However, if the muscular weakness is, in fact, due to a worsening of the disease, the clinical situation will get worse, and alternative treatment may be necessary.

SYSTEMIC LUPUS ERYTHEMATOSUS

Systemic lupus erythematosus is an immunologic disorder, with inflammatory lesions in multiple organ systems. Characteristically, there is a butterfly rash on the face, fever, polyarthropathy, and polyarthralgia. Pulmonary, renal, and cardiovascular involvement is also seen. There are alternating periods of remission and exacerbation. There is no known curative therapy. To suppress the inflammatory response, the safest drugs possible to prevent disability are used. Nonsteroidal anti-inflammatory drugs and antimalarials are used, with the glucocorticoids reserved for the more serious nephritis or cardiomyopathies.

SCLERODERMA

Scleroderma is characterized by skin thickening and a diffuse edema of the hands. There is also muscular weakness, weight loss, easy fatigability, musculoskeletal aches, and articular stiffness. A vascular instability, Reynaud's disease, is present in 80% of these patients. Contractures may develop due to the sclerosis of the skin.

There is no therapy to alter the course of this disease effectively. Supportive measures, such as analgesics, to reduce articular symptoms, and avoidance of cold environment, to protect against vascular instability, are used.

DEMYELINATING DISEASES

Demyelinating diseases involving the myelin sheath, generally sparing the axon, can occur in the central or peripheral nervous systems.

Multiple Sclerosis

Multiple sclerosis is a disease involving the destruction of the myelin sheath in the central nervous system. It is associated with an inflammatory response and is thought to be either autoimmune or slow-viral in origin, with a genetic susceptibility involved. This disease is more frequent in women, and onset is generally between the ages of 20 and 40. Both sensory and motor disturbances are evident, depending on the involved area of the central nervous system. Classic features of this disease are impaired vision, decreased perception of vibratory and proprioceptive stimuli, ataxia and intention tremor, weakness or paralysis of one or more limbs, and spasticity and flexor spasms. The clinical course is unpredictable. It may be episodic with variable waxings and wanings, or it may be progressive. Transient symptoms not related to exacerbation of the disease process may occur with overheating related to infection or strenuous exercise.

There is no cure and no proved therapy to decrease frequency or severity of relapses or to slow progression of the disease. Symptomatic treatment is administered in an attempt to ameliorate acute episodes. Clonazepam (Klonopin), a benzodiazepine, may be used to decrease cerebellar tremor. Spasticity or flexor spasms can be treated with dantrolene (Dantrium) or baclofen (Lioresal); however, generalized muscle weakness in nonspastic muscles may preclude use of these drugs in ambulatory patients. Glucocorticoids have been used in an attempt to shorten the duration of acute relapses, but there is no evidence that chronic treatment has any beneficial effect on the disease process. The use of immunosuppressive agents is under clinical study.

Guillain-Barré Syndrome

Guillain-Barré syndrome is an acute inflammatory neuropathy involving the peripheral nervous system. Again, demyelination with axonal sparing is the rule. Skeletal muscle weakness, including the muscles of respiration, can develop rapidly, so this disease should be regarded as a medical emergency. Respiratory status should be closely monitored. The muscular weakness is symmetrical and involves both proximal and distal muscles. Reflexes are depressed or absent. There may be autonomic nervous system involvement with flushing, orthostatic hypotension, and cardiac arrhythmias evident. Symptoms generally peak 2 to 4 weeks after onset, followed by an often dramatic improvement. The prognosis is good, with 85% achieving a complete, or nearly complete, recovery.

The causative factor in Guillain-Barré syndrome is not known. A viral infection frequently precedes occurrence of symptoms. An autoimmune mediation, although suspected, is obscure. Treatment is supportive, with plasmapheresis showing the greatest clinical benefit. Glucocorticoids are not considered effective.

PHYSICAL THERAPY NOTES

Physical therapy is very important in the overall clinical management of the myopathies. During the active phase of the inflammatory myopathies, dermatomyositis, and polymyositis, maintenance of range of motion is important to prevent contractures from developing. During this acute, active phase bed rest is required. However, complete bed rest is detrimental in the long term. With pharmacologic control of the disease processes, the main goal of physical therapy is to improve muscular strength. Continual evaluation of muscle strength by manual muscle testing is an important aspect of documenting the course of the disease and response to pharmacologic treatment, noting progressive or episodic changes.

In myasthenia gravis the muscle weakness is increased with acute exercise. Deep tendon reflexes may be normal, even in a weak muscle.

Drugs that can interfere with neuromuscular transmission are some antiarrhythmics and beta blockers. The antiarrhythmics quinidine and procainamide reduce excitability of the muscular membrane and probably also inhibit neuromuscular transmission. Beta blockers may interfere with neuromuscular transmission. Penicillamine can produce a clinical picture similar to the inflammatory myopathies. Drug-induced myopathies are generally reversible on withdrawal of the offending drug.

LEARNING OBJECTIVES

1. Explain the proposed abnormality in myasthenia gravis and how this interferes with normal muscle function.
2. Explain the rationale for the various pharmacologic treatments of myasthenia gravis (cholinesterase inhibitors, glucocorticoids, and immunosuppressives).
3. Understand the rationale for glucocorticoid treatment of the inflammatory myopathies.
4. Describe the involvement of physical therapy treatment of the inflammatory myopathies, both during the acute, active phase, and during long-term treatment.

ADDITIONAL READINGS

1. Argov Z, Mastaglia FL: Disorders of neuromuscular transmission caused by drugs. *N Engl J Med* 1979; 301:409–413.
2. Harvard CWH, Fonseca V: New treatment approaches to myasthenia gravis. *Drugs* 1990; 39:66–73.
3. Kantor FS: Autoimmunities: Diseases of 'dysregulation.' *Hosp Pract* 1988; 23(July):75–84.
4. Plotz PH, moderator: Current concepts in the idiopathic inflammatory myopathies: Polymyositis, dermatomyositis, and related disorders. *Ann Intern Med* 1989; 111:143–157.
5. Steinman L, Mantegazza R: Prospects for specific immunotherapy in myasthenia gravis. *FASEB J* 1990; 4:2726–2731.

Chapter 18

Respiratory Pharmacology

OBSTRUCTIVE AIRWAY DISEASES

Obstructive airway diseases include chronic obstructive airway disease (COPD) and asthma. Chronic obstructive airway disease is further subdivided into emphysema and chronic bronchitis. Although there are pathologic differences in these diseases, the major goal of therapy is to open the airways and to allow for more airflow. Some similar drugs are used in treatment of these diseases.

Emphysema

Emphysema is characterized by destruction of alveolar walls and loss of the elastic supportive tissue in the lungs. The loss of alveolar walls, while not altering alveolar volume, decreases the surface area available for capillary–alveolar gas exchange. The elastic tissue in the lungs helps maintain the noncartilaginous bronchioles patent, especially during expiration. With the loss of this supportive tissue, the pressure to collapse the bronchioles during expiration is greater than the pressure within them. Thus, there is increased resistance to airflow during expiration. Although emphysema is irreversible, the progression of symptoms may be limited if known insults are avoided. Cessation of smoking may be effective in limiting progression of the disease, especially in the early stages of the disease. Exposure to environmental/occupational irritants should be avoided, if possible. However, sometimes this may mean a change of occupation or location, which is not easily achieved. Avoidance of pulmonary diseases, with treatment of respiratory infections and seasonal flu vaccines, is also recommended.

Chronic bronchitis

Chronic bronchitis is defined as a persistent and productive cough for 3 months of the year for 2 consecutive years. Connective tissue thickens the bronchial wall, which also is infiltrated by inflammatory cells. Mucous gland secretions increase and airflow obstruction results from mucous plugs and collapse of the peripheral airway passages. Although there is hyperplasia and hypertrophy of the mucous-producing glands in the large airways, the major site of outflow obstruction seems to be the small airways. In the small airways there is an increase in inflammatory cells, with edema, fibrosis, mucous plugs, and an increase in smooth muscle.

Chronic bronchitis and emphysema may coexist. If emphysema predominates, dyspnea and hyperventilation are the dominant features, with minimal disturbance of blood gases and little production of sputum. If chronic bronchitis is the overriding component, the patient is hypoxic, cyanotic, and polycythemic, with production of copious amounts of sputum.

There is a familial susceptibility to COPD, with both genetic and environmental factors probably involved. Cigarette smoking is a major contributing factor to both emphysema and chronic bronchitis. Other contributing factors are air pollutants, especially ozone and particulates.

Bronchial asthma

Bronchial asthma is characterized by hypersensitivity of the airways to constriction, with an increased responsiveness of the respiratory tree to a variety of stimuli. An inflammatory reaction in the airways is, in part, responsible for the hyperresponsiveness and bronchospasm. Smooth muscle contraction, edema in the bronchial wall, and the presence of thick secretions all lead to increased airway resistance. An asthma attack is manifested by paroxysms of expiratory dyspnea and wheezing, overinflation of the lungs, and cough. The attacks are of variable duration, generally lasting minutes to hours. Between attacks, there are symptom-free periods and pulmonary function is nearly normal. Status asthmaticus is severe obstruction, with an attack continuing for days to weeks. This is considered a medical emergency and requires more aggressive therapy.

The hypersensitivity may be a nonallergic response to certain chemicals, such as sulfites used as food preservatives, to dyes, and even to certain drugs such as aspirin and propranolol (Inderal). Certain air pollutants, occupational and environmental dusts, exercise, decreased temperature, and emotions also may act as stimuli for an asthma attack. This disease in some people is of an allergic nature (IgE-mediated) with basophil and mast cell activation. The distinction between the allergic and nonallergic categories is not absolute.

Autocoids (locally acting chemicals) that seem to be involved in airway obstruction are many. Histamine is released from allergen-stimulated basophils and tissue mast cells. Histamine is also a mediator of the inflammatory response to nonspecific stimuli. Histamine, regardless of the cause of its release, causes arteriolar smooth muscle dilation, with increased capillary permeability leading to tissue edema and to constriction of bronchiolar smooth muscle. Histamine also increases gastric acid secretion. The different responses to histamine are mediated through two different classes of histamine receptors. H_1 receptors are on bronchial smooth muscle and capillary endothelial cells, whereas the H_2 receptors are responsible for gastric acid secretion. Drugs that interact with the H_2 receptors are discussed in Chapter 19.

That asthma is not due solely to histamine is demonstrated by the fact that drugs that block H_1 receptors, the so-called antihistamines, are not effective in relieving bronchial congestion and constriction. Other autocoids that have been implicated in asthma are certain leukotrienes (LTB_4, LTC_4, LTD_4, and LTE_4), which are products of the lipoxygenase pathway of arachidonic acid metabolism; thromboxane, a product of the cyclooxygenase pathway of arachidonic acid metabolism; bradykinin; and platelet activating factor. The nature and involvement of these and other substances in the inflammatory response are under investigation. New products that are more specific and with fewer side effects are currently under development and clinical testing.   .

Asthma predominantly occurs in children and young adults. The natural course of the disease is not well documented, but in most people, the frequency and/or severity of attacks decreases with age.

DRUGS USED IN TREATMENT OF OBSTRUCTIVE AIRWAY DISEASES

Airway capacitance may be improved in several ways, depending on the disease, by (1) relaxation of smooth muscle comprising the duct walls, (2) inhibition of inflammatory destruction and swelling of respiratory mucosa, and (3) elimination of mucosal secretions that clog the duct lumen. In both emphysema and chronic bronchitis, bronchodilators may be the only type of drug that is effective. In asthma, with its inflammatory component, additional anti-inflammatory agents may be needed. The effectiveness of mucolytics, used for liquefaction of the mucus, is not well documented. Maintenance of body hydration is important and probably better serves that purpose.

Bronchodilators

Beta adrenergic agonists

Stimulation of beta-2 adrenergic receptors causes bronchial smooth muscle relaxation. This action also facilitates mucociliary transport and decreases release of autocoids from the mast cells. Whether these secondary actions are mediated directly through beta-2 receptors is not known. Beta adrenergic agonists are indicated for treatment of acute exacerbations of asthma and exercise-induced bronchoconstriction. They also are indicated for relief of reversible bronchospasm of emphysema and chronic bronchitis. The beta adrenergic agonists may be used in combination with the glucocorticoids and/or theophylline. The nonspecific beta adrenergic agonists, such as epinephrine and isoproterenol, can cause cardiac stimulation. However, with the development of more specific beta-2 adrenergic agonists, cardiac stimulation is generally minimized. The beta-2 adrenergic agonists are not totally specific, and cardiac stimulation may be seen, especially at higher doses. Therefore, these drugs should be used with caution in patients with hypertension or ischemic

TABLE 18–1.

Beta Adrenergic Agonists for Oral Inhalation

Drug	Schedule	
	No. of Inhalations	Time
Mixed Beta Adrenergic Agonists		
Epinephrine (Bronkaid Mist, Primatene Mist)	1–2	Every 3 hr
Isoproterenol (Medihaler-Iso)	1–2	Every 3 hr
Beta-2 Adrenergic Agonists		
Metaproterenol (Alupent, Metaprel)	2–3	Every 3–4 hr
Albuterol (Proventil, Ventolin)	1–2	Every 4–6 hr
Terbutaline (Brethaire)	2	Every 4–6 hr
Bitolterol (Tornalate)	2–3	Every 8 hr
Isoetharine (Bronkosol)	1–2	Every 4 hr

heart disease. Isoproterenol stimulates both beta-1 and beta-2 receptors, whereas epinephrine stimulates not only beta-1 and beta-2 but also alpha receptors. Of the more selective beta-2 adrenergic agonists, albuterol (Proventil, Ventolin), terbutaline (Brethaire), and bitolterol (Tornalate) exhibit the most beta-2 specificity. The beta adrenergic agonists can be administered orally, by oral inhalation, or subcutaneously. Table 18–1 is a list of beta-2 adrenergic agonists that are administered by oral inhalation. Time to onset of relief of bronchoconstriction after oral inhalation is rapid, just a matter of minutes, and the effect lasts several hours. Oral inhalation generally causes fewer systemic side effects, if the drug is administered properly. Patient education and training are very important for proper use of the aerosols. Because they stimulate beta-2 adrenergic receptors in skeletal muscle, these drugs may cause tremors. Tolerance usually develops to this side effect, and it can be minimized by initiating treatment with a low dose and increasing the dose as treatment progresses.

Methylxanthines

The methylxanthines, such as theophylline, are direct acting bronchodilators whose mechanism of action is unknown. They are indicated for treating reversible bronchospasm of obstructive respiratory diseases. Drugs in this class also have an action to reduce diaphragmatic fatigue, which may aid in relief of dyspnea. Theophylline (Elixophylline, Slo-Phyllin) is the parent compound, and the others are derivatives of this. Generally, drugs in this class are less effective than the beta-2 adrenergic agonists and have a lower therapeutic index. The methylxanthines are administered orally as a sustained release preparation, and are metabolized by the liver. Table 18–2 lists the methylxanthines available for oral administration, and the usual therapeutic doses. However, serum concentrations should be monitored because of the low margin of safety. The plasma concentration of the methylxanthines may be increased with cigarette smoking and in combination with the H_2-receptor

TABLE 18–2.

Methylxanthines

Drug	Total Daily Dose	Times/Day
Theophylline (Elixophyllin, Slo-Phyllin)	13 mg/kg	3
Aminophylline (Mudrane, Somophyllin)	600–1,600 mg	3–4
Oxtriphylline (Choledyl)	20 mg/kg	3–4
Dyphylline (Dilor, Lufyllin, Neothylline)	60 mg/kg	4

blocker cimetidine (Tagamet), or with oral contraceptives. However, another H_2-receptor blocker, ranitidine (Zantac), does not affect the plasma concentration of the methylxanthines. Caffeine, another methylxanthine, should be omitted from the diet, because of additive effects with the therapeutic methylxanthines, especially in the central nervous, gastrointestinal, and cardiovascular systems. Adverse effects are nervousness, headache, nausea, vomiting, and anorexia. The methylxanthines may cause behavioral changes in children.

Anticholinergics

Parasympathetic nervous system stimulation and acetylcholine cause contraction of bronchiolar smooth muscle through stimulation of the muscarinic receptors on the smooth muscle. Anticholinergics could be used to block this; however, their use has been limited by side effects. The development of nonabsorbable anticholinergics administered by oral inhalation has allowed for direct bronchodilation through antimuscarinic actions. A new drug, ipratropium bromide (Atrovent), is such a nonabsorbable anticholinergic that is used as an inhalation aerosol. This drug has been approved for treatment of COPD, both chronic bronchitis and emphysema. Ipratropium is less effective than the beta-2 adrenergic agonists in treating asthma, but is equally as effective as the beta-2 adrenergic agonists in treatment of emphysema and chronic bronchitis. It is not rapidly acting, so it must be used consistently for best results. The recommended dose is two inhalations, four times a day. It is used for its local action in the bronchioles, and with little absorption, side effects are minimal. It does not cross the blood-brain barrier, so it does not cause the usual central nervous system adverse effects that are seen with other anticholinergics.

Antiallergic/anti-inflammatory agents

Chromones

Cromolyn sodium (Intal) is not a bronchodilator. It inhibits the allergen-induced secretion of histamine and other autocoids from mast cells during an IgE-mediated allergic response. It is used for prophylactic therapy of asthma and is not appropriate in treatment of acute asthma attacks. It is generally not as effective as the inhaled steroids, and is not even effective in all patients. It does, however, protect against exercise-induced asthma. For this purpose, it should be administered 1 to 15 minutes before exercise. It is generally well tolerated, except for possible irritant effects

TABLE 18–3.

Glucocorticoids for Oral Inhalation

Drug	No. of Inhalations	Times/Day
Beclomethasone (Vanceril, Beclovent)	2	3–4
Triamcinolone (Azmacort)	2	3–4
Flunisolide (Aerobid)	2	2

of the powder. Cromolyn sodium (Intal) is available as both a powder and an aerosol liquid. The recommended dose is two to three sprays, four times a day. The therapeutic effect may take weeks to fully develop. Tolerance to cromolyn does not develop. No special problems have arisen from use of this drug in children, so it may be the drug of choice in younger patients.

Glucocorticoids

The glucocorticoids are anti-inflammatory agents generally reserved for treatment in acute or chronic asthma that is not controlled by other agents. These drugs are not bronchodilators. Glucocorticoids are generally not used as sole therapy in treatment of asthma, but used in combination with a bronchodilator. Because of the attendant side effects of chronic systemic glucocorticoid use, this method of administration is generally reserved for potentially life-threatening acute episodes of severe asthma. Chronic systemic glucocorticoid use can cause special problems in children because of inhibition of growth. For a more complete discussion of chronic systemic glucocorticoid use, see Chapter 15. Oral inhalation or alternate-day therapy may reduce the risk of side effects seen with chronic glucocorticoid treatment. Oral inhalation provides effective local steroid activity with minimal systemic effects. Glucocorticoids available for oral inhalation therapy are listed in Table 18–3.

ALLERGIC RHINITIS

Allergic rhinitis, or hay fever, is characterized by sneezing, rhinorrhea, swelling of nasal mucosa, itching of eyes, and lacrimation. The offending allergen is generally plant pollen. Antihistamines (H_1 blockers) are usually effective.

Diphenhydramine (Benadryl) has been successfully used for many years in treatment of seasonal hay fever that is aggravated by a variety of allergens. However, it also has significant sedative and anticholinergic activity. Indications for diphenhydramine are allergic rhinitis and mild urticaria. Adverse reactions are sedation and drowsiness, which may be excessive, so that its daytime use may be limited.

Recently, new drugs have been developed that are not only effective H_1 blockers but also lack the significant central nervous system adverse effects of the more traditional antihistamines. This specificity of site of action probably occurs because they do not penetrate the blood-brain barrier. Terfenadine (Seldane) is a H_1-recep-

TABLE 18–4.

Antihistamines

Central Nervous System Effects	Total Daily Dose (mg)	Times/Day
Present		
Diphenhydramine (Benadryl)	75–200	3
Chlorpheniramine (Chlor-Trimeton)	16–24	4–6
Clemastine (Tavist)	3–8	1–3
Promethazine (Phenergan)	25	1
No significant effects		
Terfenadine (Seldane)	120	2
Astemizole (Hismanal)	10	1

tor blocker without significant central nervous system effects, such as drowsiness. Peak plasma levels are seen about 2 hours after oral administration, and it has a half-life of about 20 hours. It is extensively bound to plasma proteins. Its major side effects are related to the gastrointestinal tract, with nausea, vomiting, and gastrointestinal distress most frequently reported. It has no effect on appetite. Terfenadine is indicated for relief of symptoms associated with seasonal allergic rhinitis, such as sneezing, rhinorrhea, pruritus, and lacrimation. Peripheral anticholinergic effects such as dry mouth are similar to other H_1 blockers.

Astemizole (Hismanal) is another selective peripheral H_1 blocker. The absorption of this drug is decreased if taken with meals, so it should be taken on an empty stomach, at least 1 hour before, or 2 hours after, meals. It is metabolized in the liver. Appetite enhancement and weight gain are the most frequently reported side effects. The antihistamines, both with and without central nervous system adverse effects, are listed in Table 18–4.

PHYSICAL THERAPY NOTES

The inhalant drugs can be administered by means of a metered dose inhaler (MDI), with spacers used to improve delivery of the drug, or by nebulizers. The variability in the effective dose delivered to the lower respiratory tract depends on the hand–breathing coordination of the person. Children and the elderly may have more problems with inhalers. Proper instruction and training will help most people with this type of drug-delivery system.

Pharmacologic treatment of respiratory disease is not a cure. Emphysema and chronic bronchitis are frequently progressive, even with appropriate therapy. Exercise programs may be an important part of the overall treatment of COPD. Exercise tolerance is improved with aerobic exercise. A walking program is as effective as any, and compliance may be better. When there are limitations in the patient, such as age, advancement of lung disease, the presence of other underlying diseases, and motivation, the level of exercise achieved may not be sufficient to increase cardiovascular fitness. Also, any benefits gained with exercise will be readily lost with cessation of exercise. Breathing exercises, with slow inhalation and exhalation through pursed lips, may be helpful to prevent hyperventilation due to anxiety. Impairment of physical work capacity due to obstructive pulmonary disease can easily lead to deconditioning of the person, with its attendant decreases in pulmonary function. Chest physical therapy, including chest percussion, postural drainage, and coughing, is indicated for those patients with excessive secretions who cannot clear the secretions themselves.

In a healthy individual at rest, the work of breathing utilizes only a few percent of the total energy expended. With exercise, although the energy required to support the work of breathing increases, so does the total energy expended. Therefore, the energy required for the work of breathing is still only a few percent of the total energy expended. As obstruction to air flow increases, so does the work of breathing, especially with expiration. In the early stages of the disease, dyspnea, or discomfort associated with breathing, occurs only with intense exercise. As the obstructive processes continue, dyspnea occurs earlier with progressive exercise, until in severe obstruction, dyspnea occurs at rest. The severity of the obstruction and resultant dyspnea are, in part, the cause of the reduced level of physical activity.

Supplemental oxygen therapy is indicated in patients with severely low partial pressure of oxygen ($PO_2 < 60$ torr) and especially in those with signs of right-sided heart failure. Continuous oxygen therapy or nocturnal administration only are two regimens frequently used. Oxygen therapy frequently improves exercise tolerance.

Although exercise is a part of the overall treatment, some asthmas are triggered by exercise. Cold air seems to be the culprit, rather than any specific airborne entity. Administration of an oral inhalant, such as cromolyn sodium (Intal), before exercise can reduce this problem.

LEARNING OBJECTIVES

1. Understand the basic pathophysiology of bronchitis, emphysema, asthma, and allergic rhinitis. Explain the differences between these diseases and the similarities seen.
2. Explain the different actions and uses of the antiallergic agent (cromolyn sodium) and the anti-inflammatory agents in asthma.
3. Understand the pharmacology of the bronchodilators, beta-2 adrenergic agonists, methylxanthines, anticholinergics, and antihistamines.

ADDITIONAL READINGS

1. American Thoracic Society: Standards for the diagnosis and care of patients with chronic obstructive pulmonary disease (COPD) and asthma. *Ann Rev Respir Dis* 1987; 136:225–244.

2. Aubier A: Effect of theophylline on diaphragmatic muscle function. *Chest* 1987; 92:27S–31S.

3. Barnes PJ: A new approach to the treatment of asthma. *N Engl J Med* 1989; 321:1517–1527.

4. Glynn-Barnhart A, Hill M, Szefler SJ: Sustained release theophylline preparations. *Drugs* 1988; 35:711–726.

5. Insel PA, Wasserman SI: Asthma: A disorder of adrenergic receptors? *FASEB J* 1990; 4:2732–2736.

6. Mahler DA: The role of theophylline in the treatment of dyspnea in COPD. *Chest* 1987; 92:2S–6S.

7. McFadden ER: Corticosteroids and cromolyn sodium as modulators of airway inflammation. *Chest* 1988; 94:181–184.

8. Morris HG: Mechanisms of action and therapeutic role of corticosteroids in asthma. *J Allergy Clin Immunol* 1985; 75:1–13.

9. Newhouse MT, Dolovich MB: Control of asthma by aerosols. *N Engl J Med* 1986; 315:870–874.

10. Petty TL, Rollins DR, Christopher K, et al: Cromolyn sodium is effective in adult chronic asthmatics *Am Rev Respir Dis* 1989; 139:694–701.

11. Reed CE: Basic mechanisms of asthma. *Chest* 1988; 94:175–177.

12. Wasserman SI: Platelet-activating factor as a mediator of bronchial asthma. *Hosp Pract* 1988; 23(Nov):49–58.

PART VI

Digestion and Metabolism

Chapter 19

Gastrointestinal Pharmacology

Gastrointestinal problems beset most people during their lifetime. The control of the gastrointestinal system by the autonomic nervous system and the effects of many brain hormones on the intestinal tract allow for an intense interplay between the central nervous system and the gastrointestinal system. This interaction is probably responsible for abnormal gastrointestinal function in reaction to stress, emotions, and so forth. Prolonged stress could have profound control over gastrointestinal functions.

Aging takes a toll on gastrointestinal functions, with a slowing of most processes. Gastric acid and pepsin secretion both decrease with aging, as does gastric and intestinal motility. These normal aging processes, along with a more sedentary lifestyle, a low-fiber diet, and decreased perception of feces in the rectum and the need to defecate make the elderly more prone to gastrointestinal disturbances, especially constipation. Drug side effects on the gastrointestinal system also may cause disturbances in normal bowel functions.

The polypharmacy that is common among elderly patients complicates evaluation and treatment of digestive diseases. Constipation is a common symptom in the elderly. The causes are multifactorial, and include a low-fiber diet, sedentary lifestyle, medications, and disease processes that impair neural and motor control of the gastrointestinal tract.

PEPTIC ULCER DISEASE

Peptic ulcer disease is a group of ulcerative disorders of the upper gastrointestinal tract that have in common the participation of acid and pepsin in their pathogenesis, along with a breakdown in the mucosal defense. The corrosive effects of acid, the proteolytic effects of pepsin, and a decreased mucosal defense may be involved in ulcer development. The secretion of acid and pepsin are increased by a genetic predisposition, by smoking, and by stress. The major forms of ulcers are duodenal and gastric. Gastric ulcers are generally due to a loss of mucosal resistance. Patients generally have normal or low acid secretory rates. Gastric ulcers are

TABLE 19–1.

Commonly Used Antacids

Sodium bicarbonate
Aluminum hydroxide plus magnesium hydroxide (Maalox, Mylanta, Gelusil, Di-Gel)
Magnesium trisilicate
Calcium carbonate (Tums)

---

frequently caused by the nonsteroidal anti-inflammatory drugs (NSAIDs). Duodenal ulcers, on the other hand, are associated with an increased acid secretion and an enhanced gastric response. The parietal cells in the body of the fundus of the stomach secrete hydrochloric acid. Acid secretion is stimulated by gastrin and cholinergic postganglionic vagal fibers, by means of muscarinic receptors on parietal cells. Vagal stimulation increases gastric acid secretion directly by stimulating parietal cells and indirectly by stimulating release of gastrin. Histamine also plays an important, but poorly understood, role in acid secretion.

Most current therapies of ulcer disease are directed at reducing the effects of acid secretion. Increased acid secretion is thought to be responsible for ulcer development in the gastrointestinal tract. Currently available therapies include the old standby, antacids, and the newer histamine-$_2$ receptor blockers, proton pump inhibitors, antimuscarinic agents, site-protective agents, and prostaglandin analogues.

Antacids

A principal aim in treatment of peptic ulcer disease is neutralization of the gastric acid. For this, antacids are often used. Antacids are generally administered after meals and before bedtime. Table 19–1 lists many commonly used over-the-counter antacids.

Sodium bicarbonate is popular with the lay public. Its chronic use causes alkalosis, with sodium being absorbed followed by an increased renal excretion of hydrochloric acid. Because of the absorption of sodium, it is considered a systemic antacid. Antacids containing sodium are not recommended for those people on salt-restricted diets.

Aluminum hydroxide gel neutralizes hydrochloric acid. The gel itself is not absorbed, so no alkalosis develops. The onset of action is fairly slow. There is a tendency to constipation, more common in the elderly. Aluminum hydroxide gel binds phosphate and thus decreases phosphate absorption. This may cause anorexia, malaise, and muscle weakness. Phosphate depletion also may lead to demineralization of bone. This may be a disadvantage for postmenopausal women who already have a tendency to osteoporosis.

Magnesium hydroxide (milk of magnesia) neutralizes hydrochloric acid. This agent has a laxative effect and may be combined with aluminum hydroxide gel to counteract the constipating effect of that agent. Several combinations are available, such as Maalox, Mylanta, Gelusil, and Di-Gel.

Magnesium trisilicate, a slow-acting weak antacid, is often combined with aluminum hydroxide gel in antacids. This combination (Gelusil) forms silicon dioxide,

TABLE 19–2.

Histamine (H$_2$) Receptor Antagonists

Drug	Total Daily Dose (mg)	Times/Day
Cimetidine (Tagamet)	800	1
Ranitidine (Zantac)	300	1 or 2
Famotidine (Pepcid)	40	1 or 2
Nizatidine (Axid)	300	1 or 2

which coats the ulcers and protects from hydrochloric acid. Magnesium trisilicate also causes diarrhea.

Calcium carbonate, although prompt acting, may produce acid rebound. Calcium may be absorbed, which is the reason for the popularity of this as a calcium supplement (Tums). This agent may have a constipating effect.

Self-medication using over-the-counter antacids is a very common practice. These agents are not considered as medicine by many people, and thus may not be reported as medications in the patient's history. The placebo effect with the use of antacids is high. They are frequently used in doses too low to have any therapeutic effect. Because of the action of these agents in the gastrointestinal tract, there is a possibility of interaction with other orally administered drugs. Interference with drug absorption can occur when there are changes in gastric content pH or where the antacids form insoluble complexes with drugs. For this reason, other medications should be administered at least 1 hour before or 2 hours after an antacid.

Histamine-$_2$ Receptor Blockers

Histamine-$_2$ (H$_2$) receptor blockers are relatively new to the market and have rapidly become the most popularly prescribed drugs. The currently approved H$_2$ receptor blockers are listed in Table 19–2.

Cimetidine (Tagamet), by blocking H$_2$ receptors, prevents the histamine-triggered release of acid from the gastric parietal cells. This agent is rapidly absorbed after oral administration. Antacids are reported to interfere with its absorption, so simultaneous administration is not recommended. Cimetidine and the antacid should be taken 1 to 2 hours apart, as discussed in the preceding section. About half the absorbed dose is metabolized in the liver to inactive metabolites, and the other half is excreted unchanged by the kidneys. Because cimetidine is metabolized by the liver microsomal enzyme system, metabolism is accelerated by the presence of phenobarbital. The elimination half-life in young adults is about 2 hours. With increasing age, the elimination half-life increases. The half-life also increases with kidney and liver impairment. With advanced kidney impairment, the half-life may double. With liver impairment, the half-life may increase to 10 times normal. Cimetidine itself, through effects on the liver microsomal enzyme system, reduces metabolism of other drugs metabolized by this system, such as warfarin (Coumadin), phenytoin (Dilantin), propranolol (Inderal), chlordiazepoxide (Librium), diazepam (Valium), and the tricyclic antidepressants, with the potential of increasing their concentrations in plasma. Other agents not metabolized by the microsomal enzyme system may be substituted. For instance, there is no interaction between the beta blocker atenolol (Tenormin) and cimetidine. The other H_2-receptor blockers listed in Table 19–2 do not appear to have an effect on the mircosomal enzyme system at the recommended doses, and may be substituted for cimetidine.

Cimetidine is generally well tolerated, with infrequent side effects. With concurrent decreased renal function or in the elderly, there may be central nervous system effects, such as mental confusion, agitation, or drowsiness. Drowsiness, however, may occur in the absence of renal dysfunction. It does have antiandrogenic actions that may be seen as gynecomastia and impotence, which usually disappear with continued treatment.

Proton Pump Inhibitors

This is a new class of drugs that directly inhibits gastric acid secretion. Omeprazole (Prilosec) is the first approved drug of this class. It is a direct inhibitor of the $H^+K^+ATPase$ enzyme, the acid pump on the parietal cells. Both basal and stimulated gastric acid secretion are inhibited. It is indicated for the short-term treatment of refractory symptomatic gastroesophageal reflux disease. The standard oral dose is 20 mg, once daily. Currently, it is not approved for use in peptic ulcer disease; however, that approval may be forthcoming. Omeprazole is rapidly metabolized in the liver to inactive products, with an elimination half-life of 30 to 90 minutes. The half-life increases slightly with age. This drug is generally well tolerated with no clinically significant adverse effects. The most frequently reported adverse effects are diarrhea, nausea, dry mouth, dizziness, and headache. Its safety and efficacy with long-term therapy have not been fully evaluated. Omeprazole inhibits the liver microsomal enzyme system, so interaction with other drugs metabolized by this system, such as phenytoin (Dilantin), diazepam (Valium), warfarin (Coumadin), phenobarbital (Luminal), and carbamazepine (Tegretol), could be expected. Omeprazole prolongs the elimination of these drugs, so their doses may need to be reduced. There are no reported adverse effects related to the central nervous, cardiovascular, or respiratory systems.

Antimuscarinics

Anticholinergics selected for their antimuscarinic actions have been used to decrease motility in the gastrointestinal tract, with variable results. At much higher than recommended doses they also will decrease secretory activity. These agents are used with diet, antacids, and H_2-receptor blockers in treatment of peptic ulcer disease. They also are used to treat spastic gastrointestinal conditions such as hypermotility, mild ulcerative colitis, and gastritis. The adverse effects are dose related, antimuscarinic effects, such as dry mouth, tachycardia, urinary retention, and blurred vision. At high doses, central nervous system stimulation may be seen.

Pirenzepine is a more specific antimuscarinic agent. It shows a greater specificity in decreasing hydrochloric acid secretion and with fewer side effects than other anticholinergics. The recommended total daily dose is 100 to 150 mg, divided into two or three doses.

Site-protective Agents

Recurrence of ulcers after therapy is discontinued is common. One theory is that this recurrence is associated with the presence of a bacteria, *Helicobacter pylori*. Pepto-Bismol, which contains bismuth subsalicylate, seems to reduce bacterial infestation and ulcer recurrence. Smoking is also associated with ulcer recurrence.

Sucralfate (Carafate) is effective in treatment of peptic ulcer disease and in preventing relapse. It forms a complex that adheres to the ulcer surface and protects it from further chemical attack. There is minimal systemic absorption, so the effect is presumed to be local. For treatment of ulcers, sucralfate should be administered four times a day: 1 hour before meals and at bedtime. Treatment should be continued for 4 to 8 weeks. Following healing, maintenance therapy of twice a day treatment should be instituted to prevent recurrence of ulcers. This agent decreases absorption of cimetidine (Tagamet), digoxin, and phenytoin (Dilantin), so administrations should be separated by 2 hours. Also, antacid administration should be separated by 30 to 60 minutes. Site-protective agents, such as bismuth and sucralfate, have no influence on gastric activity, and are minimally absorbed.

Prostaglandin Analogues

Gastric ulcers associated with NSAID use may be seen in 15% to 25% of users. This is thought to be due to the inhibition of prostaglandins that are protective to the gastric tissue. Misoprostol (Cytotec) is a synthetic analogue of prostaglandin E_1 that has been approved for prevention of NSAID-related gastric ulcers. Prostaglandin analogues are better cotherapy than are antisecretory drugs. Although misoprostol is absorbed from the gastrointestinal tract, it may have a direct topical action on the gastric mucosa. Misoprostol has both antisecretory and mucosal protective actions; both basal and stimulated gastric acid secretion are inhibited. It also increases the secretion of bicarbonate and mucus. It does not interfere with NSAID treatment of arthritis and should be taken for the duration of NSAID treatment. The usual total daily dose is 400 to 800 μg, taken in divided doses. Side effects are diarrhea and cramps, which are usually transient and may respond to a reduced dose. These side effects also can be reduced by administration of the drug with meals and before bedtime, and by avoiding magnesium-containing antacids.

Misoprostol should not be administered to pregnant women because of its stimulatory effects on uterine smooth muscle. It may endanger fetal viability or induce miscarriage.

TABLE 19–3.

Laxatives

Drug	Total Daily Dose	Schedule
Stimulants		
Bisacodyl (Dulcolax)	10–15 mg	Before bedtime
Phenolphthalein (Medilax, Modane)	30–200 mg	Before bedtime
Lubricants		
Mineral oil, olive oil	—	—
Bulk laxatives		
Psyllium (Metamucil, Mucilose)	1 tsp in 8 oz liquid	1–3 times/day

CONSTIPATION

Laxatives and cathartics are used for the short-term treatment of constipation. These agents are widely used and misused by the lay public. Laxatives produce a soft-formed stool over a protracted period, whereas cathartics produce a prompt fluid evacuation. The various classes include stimulants, lubricants, bulk, saline, and fecal softening agents (Table 19–3).

Stimulant laxatives increase intestinal motor activity by a direct action. Prolonged use can lead to dependence and loss of normal bowel function. Phenolphthalein (Medilax, Modane) can lead to impaired absorption of vitamin D and calcium. The onset of action is 6 to 8 hours.

Lubricant laxatives are inert oils, such as mineral oil and olive oil. They soften fecal contents by coating them and inhibiting intestinal absorption of water. They also inhibit absorption of fat-soluble vitamins, calcium, and phosphate.

Bulk laxatives are nondigestible and nonabsorbable polysaccharides and cellulose derivatives that dissolve or swell in intestinal fluids. There is a lag time of 12 to 24 hours, or up to 36 hours, before an effect is seen. They facilitate passage of the fecal mass and stimulate peristalsis. Psyllium (Metamucil, Mucilose) is used in the management of chronic constipation. These agents may bind drugs in the gastrointestinal tract, such as anticoagulants, digoxin, and salicylates, and decrease their absorption.

DIARRHEA

Antidiarrheals are used in treatment of acute diarrhea of an inflammatory nature (Table 19–4). Kaolin (hydrated aluminum silicate) and pectin (a complex carbohydrate) are combined in Kaopectate. Kaolin adsorbs toxins, bacteria, and other noxious substances. It also adds solid matter and improves fecal consistency. Pectin provides a protective coating to irritated gastric mucosa and acts as an absorbent. There are no clinically significant adverse effects.

Bismuth subsalicylate (Pepto-Bismol) can be used for mild to moderate diarrhea. Because it contains salicylate, it should not be administered concurrently with aspirin, or to persons who should not take aspirin, for example, those on anticoagulants.

TABLE 19–4.

Antidiarrheals

Drug	Total Daily Dose; Schedule
Kaolin and pectin (Kaopectate)	3–6 tbsp; after every bowel movement
Bismuth subsalicylate (Pepto-Bismol)	2 tbsp; repeat to maximum of four doses
Diphenoxylate and atropine (Lomotil)	2 tsp; four times daily
Loperamide (Imodium)	4 mg, then 2 mg; after each bowel movement, to 16-mg maximum

Antiperistaltics are useful in treating inflammatory intestinal disorders. These synthetic opioids are effective and prompt acting. Diphenoxylate with atropine (Lomotil) decreases gastrointestinal motility. It has a half-life of 7 to 8 hours. This drug is chemically related to the narcotics. It is a controlled substance with presumed abuse potential. Thus, it may potentiate central nervous system depression if used with barbiturates, tranquilizers, and alcohol. Overdose may cause severe respiratory depression. It also may interact with the monoamine oxidase inhibitors and precipitate a hypertensive crisis.

Loperamide (Imodium) prolongs intestinal transit time, decreases volume, and increases the bulk of the fecal mass. It has a half-life of about 10 hours. Hypersensitivity to this drug may develop. Other side effects are abdominal pain and distention, nausea, and vomiting. This drug does not enter the central nervous system; thus it has no abuse potential.

PHYSICAL THERAPY NOTES

Gastrointestinal distress can interfere with a person's sense of well-being and, thus, interfere with optimal physical therapy treatment. Constipation is a common symptom in the elderly. The causes are multifactorial, with a low-fiber diet, sedentary lifestyle, medication side effects, and other disease processes as contributing factors. These, plus normal aging, can interfere with normal neural and motor functions of the gastrointestinal system. Ambulation should be encouraged to promote bowel regularity.

LEARNING OBJECTIVES

1. Describe the factors that influence ulcer development.
2. Understand the mechanism of gastric ulcer development from the use of NSAIDs.
3. Describe the different sites of action of the various classes of drugs used to treat peptic ulcer disease.

4. Understand the various factors contributing to constipation, and the actions of the drugs used to treat this symptom.

ADDITIONAL READINGS

1. Feldman M, Burton ME: Histamine-$_2$-receptor antagonists. Parts I and II. *N Engl J Med* 1990; 323:1672–1680; 1749–1755.
2. Gerbino PO, Gans JA: Antacids and laxatives for symptomatic relief in the elderly. *J Am Geriatr Soc* 1982; 30:S81–S87.
3. Lauritsen K, Laursen LS, Rask-Madsen J: Clinical pharmacokinetics of drugs used in the treatment of gastrointestinal diseases. Parts I and II. *Clin Pharmacokinet* 1990; 19:11–31; 94–125.
4. Shamburek RD, Farrar JT: Disorders of the digestive system in the elderly. *N Engl J Med* 1990; 322:438–443.
5. Soll AH: Pathogenesis of peptic ulcer and implications for therapy. *N Eng J Med* 1990; 322:909–916.

Chapter 20

Drugs Used in Treatment of Diabetes Mellitus

Insulin is a hormone secreted by the beta cells of the islets of Langerhans in the pancreas. Its action is to increase cellular uptake of glucose and amino acids, which are then utilized for cellular synthesis of glycogen, fatty acids, and proteins. Its secretion is stimulated by increased concentrations of glucose and certain amino acids in the blood. As insulin exerts its action to increase uptake and incorporation of glucose and amino acids within the cell, the blood levels of these substrates decrease. This decrease in blood glucose then inhibits insulin secretion. Thus, insulin secretion is associated with feeding and absorption of nutrients, and its actions allow for storage of nutrients that can be released and utilized by the body in times of fasting.

Some organs, such as the central nervous system, are not dependent on insulin for glucose uptake. Glucose uptake by the nervous system is dependent on the blood glucose level.

Glucagon is another hormone secreted from the pancreas, but from a different cell type, the alpha cells of the islets of Langerhans. Glucagon, in many ways, is opposed to insulin. It is secreted in response to a decreased blood glucose, and its actions are to increase liver gluconeogenesis and glycolysis. The importance of this hormone is to maintain blood glucose during times of fasting.

Diabetes mellitus is a disease in which insulin is either not present or is not appropriately secreted or acting. Diabetes is classified into two types, type I, formerly called juvenile-onset, is due to lack of insulin secretion. This also is called insulin-dependent diabetes mellitus (IDDM), or ketosis-prone. This is probably of an acquired autoimmune nature with genetic susceptibility, followed by an environmental insult, such as a virus. Induction of an immune response is then followed by destruction of the beta cells. The genetic predisposition probably is permissive rather than causal. This type of diabetes causes weight loss, polyuria, and polydipsia as its major symptoms.

Type II diabetes, formerly called maturity or adult-onset, is caused by either a lack of appropriate response to the insulin that is secreted or a lack of appropriate secretion of insulin in response to stimuli. This is not caused by a lack, per se, of insulin. In fact, the blood levels of insulin may be higher than normal. This is frequently associated with obesity. Obesity is a known risk factor for the development of type II diabetes. This also may be referred to as non-insulin-dependent diabetes mellitus (NIDDM) or ketosis-resistant. A variant of NIDDM is maturity-onset diabetes of the young (MODY).

Diagnosis of diabetes includes appropriate laboratory tests for blood levels of insulin and glucose. An oral glucose tolerance test (OGTT) is indicated for a more definitive diagnosis than can be obtained from just a fasting blood glucose level.

Diabetics are susceptible to complications, such as neuropathy, nephropathy, retinopathy, and premature atherosclerosis. Whether these are due to poor glycemic control or are part of the disease process itself is not known. Yet, most clinicians will agree that good control of glycemia will decrease morbidity and mortality from diabetic complications. Diabetics experience the same type of atherosclerosis as nondiabetics; however, they experience it earlier and more extensively. Diabetics also show evidence of small vessel disease, microangiopathy.

The neuropathy can manifest as peripheral polyneuropathy, with numbness, paresthesias, severe hyperesthesias, and pain, which is often worse at night. Early signs of neuropathy are absent stretch reflexes and loss of vibratory sense. Autonomic neuropathy is evident in the gastrointestinal tract, causing esophageal dysfunction with difficulty in swallowing, delayed gastric emptying, constipation, and diarrhea. Also, autonomic neuropathy may interfere with the cardiovascular reflexes, such as the baroreceptor reflex, and cause orthostatic hypotension.

The combination of vascular disease and neuropathy can cause serious foot problems in diabetics. Because of the neuropathy, the patient may not feel pain from a cut, abrasion, or other injury. The decreased circulation due to vascular problems impedes healing. Amputation of the foot may be the only treatment for recurrent nonhealing foot ulcers if infection has spread to bone and soft tissues of the whole foot.

Treatment of type I diabetes mellitus requires replacement of insulin. Treatment of type II, since insulin may not be lacking, may be with diet and/or an oral hypoglycemic. Insulin also may be used in type II diabetics who do not attain normal blood glucose levels with diet and an oral hypoglycemic.

INSULINS

Insulin must be administered by injection, as it is a protein and is readily digested in the intestinal tract. The currently marketed insulins are either synthesized by recombinant DNA technology or isolated from slaughterhouse animal pancreata. Pork insulin differs from human at one amino acid residue, and beef differs from human at three amino acid residues. By recombinant DNA technology, insulin is produced that has the same amino acid sequence as human insulin. This should decrease allergic reactions and decrease antibody production. Two types of antibodies can be produced against nonhuman insulin. IgE antibodies are responsible for the

TABLE 20–1.

Insulin Preparations

Type	Onset of Action	Duration of Action (hr)
Rapid-acting		
Insulin Injection	30–60 min	6–8
Regular insulin		
Regular Iletin		
Prompt Insulin Zinc Suspension	90 min	16
Semilente insulin		
Semilente Iletin		
Intermediate-acting		
Isophane Insulin Suspension	90 min	24
NPH insulin		
NPH Iletin		
Insulin Zinc Suspension	2½ hr	24
Lente insulin		
Lente Iletin		
Long-acting		
Extended Insulin Zinc Suspension	4 hr	36
Ultralente insulin		
Ultralente Iletin		
Protamine Zinc Insulin Suspension	4 hr	36
Protamine, zinc, and Iletin		

allergic reactions to insulin. IgG antibodies bind insulin but do not produce an allergic reaction. The IgG-insulin complex prevents insulin from exerting its actions. This causes a type of insulin resistance. Most people using insulin that has been isolated from slaughterhouse animals have some level of IgG insulin antibodies.

Insulin preparations are classified according to onset, duration, and intensity of action. The available insulin preparations are listed in Table 20–1. The duration and intensity of action depend on the dose: the higher the dose, the greater the intensity of action and the longer the duration of action. In renal failure there is decreased clearance of insulin, which produces a greater peak response and a longer duration of action.

The rapid-acting insulins are Insulin Injection and Prompt Insulin Zinc Suspension. Insulin in these preparations is rapidly absorbed from the subcutaneous injection site, has an onset of action of about an hour, and a duration of action of 6 to 8 hours, depending on the amount injected. The intermediately active preparations include Isophane Insulin Suspension and Insulin Zinc Suspension. These preparations have an onset of action of about 1 to 1½ hours and a duration of action of 18 to 24 hours. The preparations with a longer duration of action include Extended Insulin Zinc Suspension and Protamine Zinc Insulin Suspension. These have an onset of about 4 to 6 hours and a duration of 24 to 36 hours. A premixed preparation of 70% NPH (intermediate duration) and 30% regular (short duration) also is available.

The major side effect from insulin is hypoglycemia. This results principally from improper dosing, both amount and schedule, and inattention to dietary schedule and exercise regime. Once a dose of insulin has been injected, it continues to act until it is metabolized. Therefore, food intake must be adjusted to prevent hypoglycemia from developing. This is more important with the longer acting preparations.

The diabetic patient detects hypoglycemia from adrenergic symptoms, such as sweating, nervousness, tremor, and palpitations. If the hypoglycemia is not corrected, and progresses, central nervous system symptoms, such as confusion, abnormal behavior, loss of consciousness, and convulsions, can occur.

Fever increases the insulin requirement. There is a general increase in metabolism due to the higher temperature, which is possibly responsible for the increased insulin need. Also, insulin resistance occurs with infections. The increased insulin requirement in stress is probably related to secretion of counterregulatory hormones. This is also the mechanism of insulin resistance seen with glucocorticoid use.

A paradoxical reaction to too much insulin is posthypoglycemia hyperglycemia (Somogyi effect). This may be more common than previously thought. It is due to insulin-induced hypoglycemia initiating the hormonal responses that are necessary to counteract the initial hypoglycemia. The patient becomes temporarily out of glycemic control because the effect of the administered insulin is antagonized. This is treated by reducing the insulin dose.

Some degree of insulin resistance is usually present in diabetes. In type II diabetics, insulin resistance is probably part of the disease itself. In insulin-using diabetics, severe insulin resistance is defined as a greater than 200 units/day insulin requirement. Insulin resistance is frequently associated with insulin antibodies. However, this immune-mediated insulin resistance is less prevalent now with the improved purity of the insulins and with the availability of human insulin. This definition of insulin resistance is probably high, because the normal secretion rate is about 40 units/day. Insulin resistance may be associated with obesity, glucocorticoid use, infections, and stress.

Insulin allergy refers to the presence of IgE antibodies. This allergic reaction can produce anaphylactic shock. Insulin allergy is treated by desensitization to insulin. Special kits and instruction are available for this purpose.

ORAL HYPOGLYCEMICS

The oral hypoglycemics currently in use in the United States are chemically sulfonylureas. They do not replace insulin, but instead potentiate the effect of glucose on insulin release from the beta cells of the pancreas. They, thus, require an intact pancreas with a certain capacity for insulin secretion. These drugs also may have extrapancreatic effects such as increasing insulin receptors or increasing target organ sensitivity to insulin. These extrapancreatic effects are probably not very important because the oral agents are not effective in IDDM. All the oral agents are well absorbed from the gastrointestinal tract. However, bioavailability is better, and more

TABLE 20–2.

Oral Hypoglycemics

Drug	Duration of Action (hr)	Times/Day
Chlorpropamide (Diabinese)	24–72	1
Glipizide (Glucotrol)	16–24	1–2
Glyburide (Diabeta, Micronase)	18–24	1–2
Tolbutamide (Orinase)	6–10	2–3
Acetohexamide (Dymelor)	12–18	2
Tolazamide (Tolinase)	16–24	1–2

consistent, if they are taken about 30 minutes before a meal, rather than with a meal. The oral hypoglycemics are listed in Table 20–2.

Most side effects (i.e., hypoglycemia) are from overdosage. The longer acting agents, such as chlorpropamide (Diabinese), are more likely to cause long-lasting and severe hypoglycemia. This can be particularly a problem, when the hypoglycemia seems to last longer than the expected clearance of the drug. Generally, these agents are well tolerated. Less than 0.1% experience dermatologic (rashes, pruritis) and hematologic (hemolytic anemia, bone marrow aplasia) symptoms. About 1% to 3% will experience gastrointestinal symptoms (nausea, vomiting, dyspepsia). Chlorpropamide can cause an unusual reaction in some patients. This is called chlorpropamide alcohol flush and results in a rapid and visible flushing of the upper torso, neck, and face after consuming an alcoholic beverage. This reaction has been attributed to an Antabuse-like action, although generally not as severe. These susceptible individuals generally do not stop drinking alcohol but rather discontinue the chlorpropamide. They can generally be switched to another agent for control of blood glucose. Another reaction to chlorpropamide is similar to an inappropriate secretion of antidiuretic hormone. This is seen in 4% to 5% of patients taking chlorpropamide and causes a dilutional hyponatremia. This is more likely to occur in those with impaired volume control, such as in congestive heart failure.

All the oral hypoglycemics, except acetohexamide, are inactivated in the liver. Acetohexamide itself is a pro-drug and is activated by the liver. Therefore, liver disease can cause alterations in metabolism of all the oral hypoglycemics.

There are possible drug interactions between the oral hypoglycemics and other drugs. Use of these drugs is not always contraindicated because therapeutic doses generally do not cause a problem and the hypoglycemic dose can be changed. Alcohol, in the fasting state, suppresses gluconeogenesis, causing hypoglycemia, and producing an additive effect on the hypoglycemics. Salicylates, in large anti-inflammatory doses, have a direct hypoglycemic action and may potentiate the actions of the hypoglycemics. Dicumarol, phenylbutazone, sulfonamides, and monoamine oxidase inhibitors may prolong or enhance the action of the oral hypoglycemics by affecting drug metabolism, causing hypoglycemia. The thiazides and beta blockers reduce the efficacy of the oral hypoglycemics. Because the incidence of cardiovascular disease is increased in diabetics, these agents are likely to be prescribed together.

Treatment of diabetes mellitus, either type I or type II, requires meticulous attention to diet and exercise in addition to the pharmacologic treatment. Once the glucose-lowering agent, either insulin or an oral hypoglycemic, is administered, its glucose-lowering effect lasts as long as the agent is present. Therefore, to prevent too much glucose lowering, diet and exercise must be appropriate for the amount of the drug administered. Oral hypoglycemics are less likely to produce hypoglycemia than insulin. However, when hypoglycemia does occur in response to an oral agent, it is usually severe and prolonged.

Exercise is very important to the total treatment of diabetes mellitus. Exercise causes a non-insulin-dependent glucose uptake. In nondiabetics, exercise thus causes a decrease in insulin secretion. However, in diabetics, this normal control cannot happen. The patient should either reduce the dose of insulin if he or she knows that exercise will occur or else consume a glucose-containing food in order to provide substrate for the insulin, and thus prevent hypoglycemia from developing. Another aspect of exercise is important to those taking insulin. Exercise increases blood flow to the exercising muscles. If insulin had been administered by injection to that area, the increased blood flow will remove insulin faster from its site of injection. Insulin administered before exercise should be injected into a nonexercising extremity or into the abdomen. Exercise is beneficial to diabetics in many ways, and should not be neglected as part of the total treatment of the disease. Exercise decreases low-density lipoprotein and raises high-density lipoprotein. Because diabetics are at increased risk for microvascular and macrovascular disease, an improvement in blood lipid profiles would be beneficial. Also, in those who are overweight, exercise may be a part of a proper weight loss program. In many type II overweight diabetics, weight loss may be associated with a lessening of the diabetes, due to an improved insulin sensitivity. This can result in a decrease in the dose of the antidiabetic agent, either insulin or oral hypoglycemic.

PHYSICAL THERAPY NOTES

Because of the multiple system involvement in diabetes mellitus, these patients can present to the physical therapist with a multitude of problems. Because of the poor circulation to the lower extremities, open wounds are slow in healing. Sores may develop more frequently in diabetics because of peripheral neuropathy, with decreased sensation. Thus, the sores may be quite large before the person notices them. Meticulous foot care is essential. Correct fitting shoes can prevent pressure sores from developing. Going barefooted is contraindicated because of the likelihood of foot injury. Prevention is overall much easier than treatment.

Peripheral neuropathy also may lead to a loss of proprioception. Precise movement and placement of feet during ambulation may be lacking. This can lead to apparent gait deviations.

Autonomic neuropathy can cause a blunting or slowing of the baroreceptor reflex. This can cause postural hypotension. Avoidance of rapid changes in posture are necessary to prevent serious injury occurring from falls and fractures. Exercise improves circulation, improves glucose tolerance, and may improve lipid profiles.

LEARNING OBJECTIVES

1. Understand the physiologic actions of insulin, especially regarding carbohydrate, fat, and protein metabolism.
2. Describe the differences between type I (juvenile onset) and type II (adult onset) diabetes, as related to causes, age at onset, and type of treatment.
3. Explain the overall goal of treatment of an insulin-dependent diabetic patient, and the interactions of insulin treatment with diet and exercise. Describe the different types of available insulin, both as to onset and duration of action.
4. Describe the actions of the oral hypoglycemics in non-insulin-dependent diabetic patients.
5. Explain the importance, in treated diabetics, of diet and exercise with diabetic therapy, either insulin or oral hypoglycemics.

ADDITIONAL READINGS

1. Breidahl HD: What patients with diabetes want to know about their therapy. *Drugs* 1980; 19:135–140.
2. Gerich JE: Oral hypoglycemic agents. *N Engl J Med* 1989; 321:1231–1245.
3. Jarrett RJ: Cardiovascular disease and hypertension in diabetes mellitus. *Diab Metab Rev* 1989; 5:547–558.
4. Melander A, Bitzén P-O, Faber O, et al: Sulphonylurea antidiabetic drugs. *Drugs* 1989; 37:58–72.
5. Moller DE, Flier JS: Problems of insulin resistance. *Hosp Pract* 1988; 23(Oct):83–96.
6. O'Byrne S, Feely J: Effects of drugs on glucose tolerance in non-insulin-dependent diabetics. Parts I and II. *Drugs* 1990; 40:6–18; 203–219.
7. Zawada ET: Metabolic considerations in the approach to diabetic hypertensive patients. *Am J Med* 1989; 87(suppl 6A):34S–38S.
8. Zinman B: The physiologic replacement of insulin. *N Engl J Med* 1989; 321:363–370.

PART VII

Geriatrics

Chapter 21

Pharmacology and the Geriatric Population

The elderly constitute the most rapidly growing segment of the population. There is an increased awareness of, and concern for, health problems in this age group, especially related to the association between aging and the increase in frequency and number of diseases. There is an increased consumption of drugs, both total amount of drugs and number of different drugs, that reflects the multiple pathologic states present in this age group. Both the increase in diseases and the increase in number of drugs taken cause an increase in morbidity, with subsequent disability. There are changes in physiology associated with aging. Basically, there is a decreased reserve of most systems. With advancing age, compensatory mechanisms are often delayed or insufficient. Impaired function may be evident only when the system has been stressed, such as in the presence of a disease. In general, the elderly are more sensitive to actions and side effects of many drugs. With careful prescribing of drugs and monitoring of the patient, many adverse reactions can be minimized. Because of increased incidence of chronic diseases and multiple health problems of the elderly, people in this age group are more likely to be subject to "polypharmacy," the prescribing of multiple drugs. This may cause drug-drug interactions that would not be seen with use of a drug by itself. The risk of adverse reactions increases with every drug added. Multiplicity of treatments causes more adverse drug reactions than aging itself.

Some cellular and organ changes that occur with aging have effects on both the pharmacokinetics and pharmacodynamics of many drugs. Alterations in pharmacokinetics may increase the availability of a drug. The elderly may respond differently to many drugs due to age-associated changes in liver and kidney function. With aging there is a decrease in liver blood flow and metabolism. This can lead to an increased half-life of drugs cleared by the liver. On the other hand, drugs that are activated by the liver may show a decreased response. In the kidney, decreases in renal blood flow, glomerular filtration rate, and tubular secretion can increase the half-life of drugs eliminated by the kidney.

The shift in body mass from lean or muscle tissue to fat tissue associated with aging causes a decreased total body water content. Water-soluble drugs thus have a decreased volume of distribution, resulting in an increased plasma concentration. Digoxin is an example of a drug whose plasma concentration can be affected by this mechanism. On the other hand, with the shift in body composition, the percent of body weight as fat tissue increases. Lipid-soluble drugs have a greater volume of distribution and an increase in their apparent half-life. Calcium blockers fall in this category. With the elderly, careful monitoring of drug action, side effects, and dosage adjustment, with frequent reassessment, are required to minimize side effects. Drugs that are particularly troublesome in the elderly are those with long half-lives, especially those that require hepatic metabolism.

Altered sensitivity to certain drugs in the elderly may be due to changes in end-organ responsiveness. Autonomic dysfunction or failure seen in the elderly, whether due to aging or as part of a disease process, is most likely associated with a decrease in beta receptor sensitivity. The baroreceptor reflex is decreased, presenting as a decreased or absent heart rate response to hypotension. With beta receptor insensitivity, the response to both beta agonists and beta antagonists is decreased. The elderly are more sensitive to drugs with anticholinergic activity. Urinary retention, blurred vision, orthostatic hypotension, and mental confusion are more likely to occur as anticholinergic side effects in this age group.

ADVERSE EFFECTS OF SPECIAL CONCERN IN THE ELDERLY

Impaired balance

Decreased function in certain sensory systems are likely to lead to balance disturbances that can ultimately cause decreased independent ambulation. Visual impairment itself or poor adjustment to corrective lenses, especially bifocals, can have a detrimental effect on balance. Loss of proprioceptive sense, especially in the lower limbs, and deterioration of vestibular reflexes are likely to impair balance reactions. Drugs which cause dizziness, sedation, or hypotension, including alcohol, can exacerbate any balance deficiencies and decrease gait efficiency. Just the fear of a possible fall can inhibit progress to independent ambulation.

Sedation

Drugs with sedating actions, especially those with the potential to impair motor and cognitive function, are a definite problem in the elderly. Falls and/or accidents may be precipitated by drugs that cause sedation, dizziness, or orthostatic hypotension.

Sedative-hypnotics are overused in the treatment of subjective reports of insomnia. A prolonged duration of action may lead to daytime sedation, with impairment of mental and physical function. Changes in sleep patterns with aging are considered normal, and should be of no concern. Lifestyle and dietary habits may, however, accentuate these changes, causing disturbing symptoms, such as insomnia or nighttime wakening. Daytime napping can hinder falling asleep at bedtime. For bedridden patients, this is a particular problem. The elderly are generally more sensitive to central nervous system stimulatory effects of caffeine in coffee, tea, and soft drinks. Also, the diuretic effect of caffeine can cause nighttime waking for trips to the bathroom. Nonpharmacologic treatment, such as changes in before-bedtime habits, are more effective in the long term, definitely safer, and pose fewer problems of increasing disability.

Depression

Lack of motivation, decreased interest in surroundings, and lack of cooperation are related to depression. Depression is more common in the elderly and may be associated with a disease or with use of a drug. Antihypertensive drugs, such as the central alpha agonists, clonidine (Catapres) and methyldopa (Aldomet), and the direct acting vasodilator hydralazine (Apresoline) may cause depression. Propranolol (Inderal) has been associated with depression. Although depression is associated with Parkinson's disease, it also is associated with levodopa therapy. Digitalis can cause depression, as can diazepam and other sedatives.

Lethargy, which is defined as subjective feelings of apparent general weakness, may be related to depression or evidence of underlying disease, such as pulmonary disease, heart failure, or vascular insufficiency. In addition to the sensory deficiencies mentioned earlier, decreased muscle strength from deconditioning will alter gait efficiency.

Mental confusion

The use of sedatives, hypnotics, antianxiety agents, and antipsychotic drugs in the elderly can cause mental confusion or disorientation and impaired mental function. Mental confusion is also a possible adverse effect from drugs with anticholinergic actions. Antihistamines, such as diphenhydramine in over-the-counter cold remedies and in sleep-inducing agents, pose a noteworthy problem, as their use may not be closely monitored. Antipsychotic drugs, especially chlorpromazine (Thorazine), have serious anticholinergic actions. Of the tricyclic antidepressant drugs, amitriptyline (Elavil), is the most anticholinergic. Disopyramide (Norpace), a class Ia antiarrhythmic agent, is highly anticholinergic. The antiparkinson drugs, both the anticholinergic drugs and the dopaminergic drugs, can cause confusion and delirium. Mental confusion also can be caused by cimetidine (Tagemet) and digitalis.

Mental confusion can lead to a vicious cycle in drug administration, resulting in poor compliance. There can be either incomplete control of the disease because of decreased drug intake, or increased adverse drug reactions owing to increased drug intake.

Skeletal muscular weakness

Although skeletal muscular weakness is caused by bed rest and inactivity, it can be related to medical problems such as cardiovascular, pulmonary, or musculo-skeletal disease. Certain drugs also are known to cause muscular weakness. Beta blockers (probably by blocking beta receptors in skeletal muscle) and diuretics (by causing hypokalemia) can lead to muscular weakness. Sedatives also can lead to muscular weakness.

Anticholinergic effects

Antimuscarinic side effects from drugs may develop gradually and may mimic changes thought to be associated with aging, such as dry mouth, constipation, and memory loss. The elderly are more sensitive to antimuscarinic side effects related to the central nervous system. This possibly results from the age-associated decrease in cholinergic activity in the central nervous system. Urinary retention, constipation, blurred vision, orthostatic hypotension, oversedation, and mental confusion can increase morbidity. The antihistamines in the over-the-counter cold remedies and sleep-inducing agents pose a particular problem, as their use may not be closely monitored. The antipsychotic drug chlorpromazine (Thorazine) is particularly anticholinergic, as is amitriptyline (Elavil), and the class Ia antiarrhythmic, disopyramide (Norpace).

DEMENTIA

Currently, dementia is defined as a clinical syndrome composed of failing memory and loss of other intellectual functions as the result of a chronic and progressive degenerative disease of the brain. It also is associated with certain behavioral abnormalities and changes in personality. Dementia may exist by itself (Alzheimer's and senile). It may be associated with other neurologic diseases, such as Huntington's chorea, Parkinson's disease, cerebrocerebellar degeneration, cerebral arteriosclerosis, or brain tumor. Other medical non-neurologic diseases, such as hypothyroidism and Cushing's disease, or nutritional deficiencies, such as pellagra, may cause dementia. Chronic drug intoxication, such as with barbiturates, alcohol, and other sedatives may cause an apparent dementia. Alzheimer's disease is the most common cause of dementia in the elderly. Although advancing age is accompanied by neuronal loss in the cerebral cortex, dementia is not an inevitable accompaniment of aging. The biochemical cause of dementia is not known; however, it is thought to be due, in part, to a cholinergic defect. With aging there is a decrease in acetylcholine in the central nervous system, and this has been associated with memory loss. Other neurotransmitter systems also are likely to be involved.

The only approved drug for treating the symptoms of dementia is Hydergine, which contains synthetic ergoloid mesylates. In some patients this drug may alleviate symptoms of dementia. In light of the cholinergic dysfunction theory, pharmacologic improvement of cholinergic transmission is under study. Tacrine (Cognex), also known as THA, is an acetylcholinesterase inhibitor. This drug is under experimental investigation concerning its efficacy in treatment of Alzheimer's disease. The limitation of this type of drug is due to the progressive nature of the disease. As the cholinergic neurons degenerate, these agents would be expected to have less and less effect. As we get a better handle on the cellular aspects of the disease, better pharmacologic agents will be developed. Under investigation also are muscarinic agonists, acetylcholine precursors, and other acetylcholinesterase inhibitors.

POSTURAL HYPOTENSION

Postural, or orthostatic, hypotension is decreased blood pressure on standing, sufficient to produce symptoms mainly related to cerebral hypoperfusion or cardiac hypoperfusion. It occurs in a significant percent of elderly people and may be a significant contributor to morbidity and mortality from falls and subsequent injury. Symptoms range from dizziness or lightheadedness to syncope. Angina may be a symptom if coronary perfusion is decreased. Transient ischemic attacks may be seen when cerebral circulation is compromised. Postural hypotension may be related to the aging process, as part of the autonomic dysfunction seen in the elderly. There is a decreased sensitivity of the baroreceptors to changes in blood pressure with aging. Certain diseases may include autonomic dysfunction among their clinical manifestations, such as parkinsonism, cerebrovascular pathology, and diabetes mellitus.

Specific drugs also contribute to the more frequent occurrence of postural hypotension in the elderly. Chlorpromazine (Thorazine), because of its alpha blocking activity; antihypertensive drugs (especially prazosin [Minipress], methyldopa [Aldomet], clonidine [Catapres], hydralazine [Apresoline], and many diuretics); amitriptyline (Elavil), because of its alpha blocking activity; levodopa; antianxiety agents; nitrates; and several over-the-counter drugs may precipitate hypotension. Other causes of postural hypotension are prolonged bed rest; volume depletion and dehydration; electrolyte imbalance, especially hypokalemia; and cardiac arrhythmias. Symptoms are generally worse in the morning, after a meal, and after exercise or a hot bath.

Nonpharmacologic management is frequently possible. There may be a need to reduce the dose of a drug or to change to a drug that has less of a hypotensive effect. The patient is advised to change positions slowly, especially on arising from bed in the morning. Sitting on the edge of the bed and moving the legs and feet with active dorsiflexion before standing up can be sufficient to prevent a fall. Avoidance of heavy meals, with more frequent smaller meals, may alleviate hypotensive reactions. Also, avoidance of hot baths and vigorous exercise resulting in vasodilation may alleviate problems. In more serious cases the person may need elevation of the head at night by 8 to 12 inches to minimize nocturnal diuresis. Graduated pressure stockings that extend to the waist improve venous return and cardiac output. Attention to adequate sodium and water intake is important to prevent dehydration and volume contraction.

Pharmacologic treatment may include fludrocortisone acetate, a synthetic mineralocorticoid that increases extracellular and plasma volumes and potentiates the norepinephrine response on vascular receptors. This drug should be used with caution, with monitoring of cardiac status, especially with regards to hypertension, congestive heart failure, and hypokalemia. Indomethacin (Indocin), an inhibitor of prostaglandin synthesis, may be effective especially in treatment of postprandial hypotension. However, this drug may cause gastrointestinal irritation. Considering the number of drugs an elderly person is possibly already taking, nonpharmacologic interventions seem the better choice, if they are effective.

In patients with postprandial hypotension, caffeine (two cups of coffee) administered before the meal may be effective. However, since habituation to coffee frequently occurs, its effects may be short lived.

PHYSICAL THERAPY NOTES

As stressed in this chapter, the elderly are not only more sensitive to actions and adverse effects of drugs, they also are more likely to be taking multiple drugs. The increased incidence of adverse drug effects among the elderly is a major health problem and a contributor to morbidity and disability. Multiple drug use also can interfere with diagnosis of medical problems.

All cases of memory loss and mental confusion are not necessarily Alzheimer's disease. In many cases, offending drugs are the culprit.

Postural hypotension is, obviously, best avoided. Just the fear of falling can inhibit progression to independent ambulation. Nonpharmacologic management may be possible. If a person has been in bed for even a few days, the upright position may not be well tolerated. Arising slowly from lying down, to side sitting, resting on elbows, with active dorsiflexion of the feet, may protect the person from sudden drops in blood pressure and cerebral perfusion. A tilt table can be used, especially with orthopedic patients, such as following hip replacement. Slowly bring the table to almost upright with frequent stops and blood pressure and heart rate checks. With any drop in blood pressure, the table can be lowered until blood pressure normalizes.

LEARNING OBJECTIVES

1. Understand the physiologic changes associated with aging that can alter the body's handling of drugs (i.e., changes in liver and kidney function).
2. Explain the physiologic changes associated with aging that can alter response to drugs (e.g., increased sensitivity to anticholinergic actions and decreased beta receptor sensitivity).
3. Describe the drugs that can have adverse effects on the central nervous system and produce sedation, depression, and mental confusion.

4. Understand the physiologic and pharmacologic causes of postural hypotension. List the drugs known to exacerbate postural hypotension.

ADDITIONAL READINGS

1. Ahmad RAS, Watson RDS: Treatment of postural hypotension. *Drugs* 1990; 39:74–85.
2. Applegate WB, Blass JP, Williams TF: Instruments for the functional assessment of older patients. *N Engl J Med* 1990; 322:1207–1214.
3. Beers MH, Ouslander JG: Risk factors in geriatric drug prescribing. *Drugs* 1989; 37:105–112.
4. Brawn LA, Castleden CM: Adverse drug reactions: An overview of special considerations in the management of the elderly patient. *Drug Safety* 1990; 5:421–435.
5. Bressler R: Multiple drug use in an elderly man. *Hosp Pract* 1987; 22(July):111–127.
6. Lipsitz LA: Orthostatic hypotension in the elderly. *N Engl J Med* 1989; 321:952–957.
7. McCormick WC, Larson EB: Pragmatism and probabilities in dementia. *Hosp Pract* 1990; 25(Dec):93–114.
8. Palmer AM, Gershon S: Is the neuronal basis of Alzheimer's disease cholinergic or glutamatergic? *FASEB J* 1990; 4:2745–2752.
9. Peters NL: Antimuscarinic side effects of medications in the elderly. *Arch Intern Med* 1989; 149:2414–2420.
10. Prinz PN, Vitiello MV, Raskind MA, et al: Geriatrics: Sleep disorders and aging. *N Engl J Med* 1990; 323:520–526.
11. Rowe JW, Kahn RL: Human aging: Usual and successful. *Science* 1987; 237:143–149.
12. Steinberg JR: Prescription drug impairment in the elderly. *Drug Therapy* 1990; 20(suppl, Aug):83–98.
13. Sudarsky L: Geriatrics: Gait disorders in the elderly. *N Engl J Med* 1990; 322:1441–1446.
14. Weber MA, Neutel JM, Cheung DG: Hypertension in the aged: A pathophysiologic basis for treatment. *Am J Cardiol* 1989; 63:25H–32H.

INDEX